Testimonials

"I feel reborn! Although more than one month has passed, the back pain has never come back."

– Toshi K., Torrance, CA – Yelp

"I have suffered from back pain for twenty years, and this method has helped tremendously. It is gentle, not painful, and is effective."

– Mery Girl, iBooks

"This book is a great way to utilize the releases he uses on me in his office while at home. They are simple and work wonders. The book is a great guide and very easy to use. If you are in pain, buy this book!"

– Vanessa – Amazon

"I have used this book to help me get out of pain! Using the releases illustrated in this book, I was able to calm down my muscle spasm and be back to normal in less than 24 hours. Try the easy-to-follow instructions in this book, be patient, and see what wonders it can accomplish!"

– Dr. J. Sullivan – Amazon

"I call him Gadi 'The Maestro' Kaufman because he is a virtuoso with his fingers on the muscles of the body! He truly is a 'nerve whisperer.'"

– C's M, Nevada City, CA – Yelp

"Gadi Kaufman was the first practitioner in twenty years to help me get free from pain. Other well-meaning and highly-trained folks tried, but this method has worked for me better than anything else. If you suffer from back pain, then buy this book. I use it all the time, and it works."

– BBRomm – Amazon

"Once you take the time to understand the true sources of your pain, these positions can change your life. I am thankful to Gadi for giving me my physically-active life back. I now do several of the key positions each day. Give it a try."

– P. Orosco – Amazon

"Seeing Gadi and doing the exercises in this book are my last resort after having tried chiropractic care, trigger point shots, shiatsu massage, physical therapy, and acupuncture. I am beginning to sleep better due to my muscles learning how to relax, and am experiencing a lessening of high night time cortisol levels. I highly recommend this book to anyone who is looking for a proven method of pain relief for tight spastic muscles."

– Anonymous – Amazon

"This guy is simply a genius. I have been seeing him for a month and am now pain free. The thing that I like the most is that he is a no-frills guy who just wants to help people."

– Richa K., Culver City, CA – Yelp.com

"Gadi is the best! The Strain Counterstrain method is the only method that works for relieving pain in my back."

– Rachel F., Irvine, CA – Yelp.com

In-Office Clients

"I had an automobile accident that resulted in two back surgeries. I worked with physical therapists for 40 years but was unable to regain complete mobility, and I suffered from chronic pain. As I aged, my mobility declined and the pain grew more aggravated. Gadi Kaufman changed everything. Today I am restored to complete mobility and am pain free. It's a miracle to be able to walk like a normal person and even play sports. Gadi Kaufman is a genius who will improve your life."

– Neil Levin, California

"The type of therapy that Gadi Kaufman uses has been a life saver for me! I've been able to stay active and play tennis after 20 years of suffering from severe muscle spasms in my upper body. I also learned how to deal with occasional muscle spasms on my own. He has changed my life and taught me how to be aware of my body and maintain good posture."

– Robin Thayer – Marina del Rey, California

"A treatment with Gadi is better than any massage. You will feel like going into a deep sleep. The technique addresses the real issue—muscles that want to relax, but can't because they are in spasm. The technique will give your body the chance to truly feel better and heal because O2 and blood can now circulate to the muscle. Don't waste your time or money anywhere else. Go see Gadi!"

– Jane Graves – Los Angeles, California, ladybugjane.com

"I am a fit, committed health professional, but two years ago I experienced so much pain in my rear end and side thighs that I couldn't function. My world revolved around my pain. 'How does one live with such pain?' was the question asked by a team of practitioners including a podiatrist, neurologist, neuro-surgeon, chiropractor, acupuncturist, physical therapist, massage therapist, and psycho therapist. All had opinions, but Gadi was the only person that said 'you don't have to' and then proceeded to alleviate my spasms and give me methods to relieve them myself. I am back in the gym, walking, biking, and doing yoga. What a relief! Thank you Gadi."

– G. McMahon RN, BSN – Calabasas, California

"I could not thank you enough for helping me get rid of my headaches following the bus accident in Rome. I had never suffered from frequent headaches in the past, but after the accident, I lived on pain killers. One visit with you relieved the pressure from my neck and the headaches were gone."

– Hanna Lidgi – Thousand Oaks, California

"I suffered from plantar fasciitis for 9 months before I went to see Gadi. The pain in my heel was constant and close to debilitating. Prior to seeking treatment from Gadi I was treated by a podiatrist and a physical therapist, neither of whom was able to help. Gadi suggested that the problem was not originating from my heel or foot, but from my calf. He treated me 6 times over the course of 3 weeks. And just like that... problem solved. Gadi's method of relief cost me a fraction of what I had already spent for unsuccessful visits elsewhere. To say it was nearly like magic is not hyperbole. Thank you, Gadi!"

– Jeff – Los Angeles, California

Do It Yourself Back Pain Relief In 90 Seconds

The pain-free approach to resetting the nervous system and releasing muscle spasms

Gadi Kaufman NMT, JSCC

http://gadibody.com

Disclaimer

This book is intended to be a helpful reference, and not a replacement for the guidance, diagnosis, treatment, and care of your physician and other health and medical professionals. For concerns about any medical condition you may have, seek the advice of a trained medical professional. The author, publisher and all associated with the creation of this book are not liable for loss, injury or damages that may occur as a result of the information and images within this book.

Medical illustrations reprinted with permission by Wolters Kluwer Brown. From Travell & Simmons', *Myofascial Pain and Dysfunction: The Trigger Point Manual* Vol. 1 and Vol. 2 Copyright © 1998 and 1992 by Wolters Kluwer Brown.

Original Illustrations by Josh Evans
Book Design and Production by Derek Padula: //derekpadula.com

For my wife Sandra and my son Ethan

The nervous system is the boss.
The muscles are the employees.

Contents

Introduction   ix

Step-by Step Guide   xix

Psoas   1

Iliacus (center)   17

Rectus Abdominus   31

Oblique (lower)   45

Iliacus (lower)   59

Oblique (upper)   83

Spinal   105

Quadratus Lumborum   127

Piriformis   141

Conclusion   153

About the Author   155

Reference Guide   157

Introduction

Do you suffer from lower back pain? Is it so bad that you can no longer live a normal life? Does it hurt to get in and out of your car or to sit at the kitchen table? Is it difficult to change position in bed without pain? Or maybe you can't bend over to pick up your kids or a bag of groceries without wincing and grabbing your lower back. People tell you to exercise, but it's too painful and you avoid walking long distances for fear of exacerbating the problem. Instead, you take every chance to lie on the floor in hopes of getting some momentary relief.

You're not alone. Did you know that one out of four Americans suffer from debilitating lower back pain?

The reason lower back pain is so common is that we live in a sedentary society. To say it simply: We sit too much. We sit in the car driving to work. We sit at the office all day because of the necessity of using a computer. Then we sit in the car driving back home. Once there, we sit at home watching television or grab a laptop and kick back into a chair. Sound familiar? All of this goes against the biomechanics of the human body. We are biomechanically designed to stand and walk, not to sit for so many hours a day.

Here in lies the dilemma for the back pain sufferer. To be healthier, you need to do more moving, walking, and standing. But if you have lower back pain, then moving, walking, and standing is not something you can do without crying out in pain.

So how do you find relief? As you know, there are many options out there today and surely you've tried them all: from pain medications to acupuncture, to chiropractic care, massage, and physical therapy or even the last resort of surgery.

Maybe one of these methods has provided you with temporary relief for short periods of time. But did your relief last? Were you able to alleviate your pain long enough to return to normal life and enjoy your daily activities?

What you don't know about lower back pain

There's no question that these other practitioners have tried with good intentions to diminish your lower back pain. And if you've been to see a massage therapist or another specialist, what you've noticed is that the work they do in treatment is focused primarily on the part of your body that feels the pain—meaning, your lower back. They go straight to the symptomatic area and massage muscles or insert tiny needles. And that seems logical, right? Well, maybe not.

In this book, you're going to learn some very important information about lower back pain that you have not been told by other practitioners.

Did you know that the majority of lower back pain does not actually originate in the lower back muscles themselves? In other words, while you feel pain in your lower back, very often, the source of your discomfort can be traced to the front of the body. Yes, that's right: In most cases the source of lower back pain can be found in the front of the body, and it then radiates from there to the lower back.

There are several muscles in the abdomen and hip area that we use to sit, stand, and walk.

One of the most important is the iliopsoas muscle. This muscle attaches to the side and front of the lower spine. From there it continues down through the inside of the hip bone and connects to the top of the thigh bone on the inside.

Naturally, these muscles get tired from over-use. And when they do, a chain reaction occurs that spells trouble for you. This is what typically happens: When your worn-out and fatigued muscles can no longer function properly, they go through a process that puts them into a spastic state called a spasm. A spasm means they are locked in a shortened position and contracted to the point where they have lost their ability to lengthen. At the same time, the body's nervous system contributes by helping to put and keep a muscle in spasm indefinitely. And while in spasm, the muscles can twist and torque the spine, cause rotation of the pelvis in several directions (usually forward and to the side), and finally lead to compression of the thigh into the hip socket on one or both sides of the body. (For more details, visit *gadibody.com* and read the article "Understanding Biomechanics.")

After all this, you are experiencing a whole lot of pain—which began in the front of the body—that has referred to the lower back and hips. And as if that isn't enough, this chain reaction causes the spinal muscles (which are on either side of the spine starting at the sacrum running all the way up to the back of the neck) to spasm as well.

The good news is that you can do something about it. And in this book, you're going to learn how by using a technique that focuses on the source of the pain which is at the front of the body. This technique is called Strain Counterstrain. A friendlier name for this technique is positional release. Although the word "strain" is included in its name, there is no straining involved. Instead, it's a passive, gentle, and stress free way to bring relief to your lower back pain. It doesn't require any spinal manipulations, uncomfortable maneuvers, or deep tissue massage. You'll do it without harsh medications or additional pain. And best of all, you can do it on your own, at home, without equipment.

Before I can teach you how to do this remarkable technique, it's important to first understand the concept behind Strain Counterstrain, which involves the body's muscular system and its nervous system.

Understanding the muscular system

Your muscles work as the cable system of the body. Some of your muscles are responsible for movement of the body, while others are tasked with holding the body up against gravity. Your bones have no ability to move on their own. The only reason they are able to move is because they are connected to muscles. The role of the muscles is to move the body in space, and if we hope to live a healthy and productive life, our muscles need to function properly.

In a perfect world, healthy muscles would contract (shorten) and stretch (lengthen) as necessary and enable you to move around with ease. You could get in and out of a chair without difficulty. You could bend down and pick up something off the floor without hesitation.

Unfortunately, we don't live in a perfect world, and the reality is that in our hectic modern lives, our bodies don't always perform the way they are naturally designed. Most of us don't use our muscular system in the most efficient way. All too often, the muscles you're supposed to use when walking down the street, or raising your leg to step into your car, or kneeling down to pick up something, are not properly engaged.

The body is hardwired to push through physical limitations and keep us moving, even in less than optimal circumstances such as these. So when a muscle is unable to do its own job, the body automatically recruits neighboring muscles to pitch in and help. And while these helper muscles do their best to comply with these requests, they can only deliver for a limited period of time. Even then, they do so at a cost. As they perform tasks they were never intended for, a burden is placed on the entire muscular system and it doesn't take long until a breakdown occurs. Some muscles become over-used while others become under-used. This leads to a muscular imbalance. Muscles become fatigued and fall into a weakened state.

Our bones are dependent on our muscles. We know that our muscles are not independent structures and they do not have a mind of their own to inform them when to engage. They do not decide on their own when to contract, lengthen, or to stay locked in a spasm. So how do our muscles know what to do?

The role of the autonomic nervous system

For any muscle to take action—whether it's healthy or unhealthy—it must receive instructions from the brain. The brain sends instructions (electric signals known as impulses) to the muscles through the nervous system, and the muscles receive these signals through sensors that are embedded in the muscle fibers.

If your muscles are functioning properly, they receive instructions to perform by contracting and stretching, and you can get where you need to without discomfort.

But when muscles are not functioning properly and they are stuck in contraction (spasm), then the whole muscular system is in chaos.

As you can see, the nervous system's role in creating a painful muscle spasm is critical. The process begins with an over-used muscle that has become fatigued, or with an over-stretched muscle which is at risk of being torn.

In order for this dysfunctional muscle to find out what it should do under these difficult circumstances, it sends a distress signal to the autonomic nervous system in the form of alpha signals. This muscle is in trouble and is reaching out to the nervous system for help. It is saying to the autonomic nervous system that there is a threat to normal activity and it is unable to engage properly. In response, the autonomic nervous system communicates to the muscle by sending gamma signals that instruct the muscle to stop functioning. And once it does stop, a spasm is created.

So far we've described how the exchange of alpha and

gamma signals begins with the muscles.

This exchange of messages can also start from the autonomic nervous system when a person is under a tremendous amount of emotional or psychological stress. Either way, this is where trouble starts and takes you down the path to a muscle spasm.

At this point we have a Catch 22 situation.

The autonomic nervous system and the spastic muscle continue sending alpha and gamma signals back and forth and the muscle cannot get out of the spastic state. Believe it or not, the autonomic nervous system's underlying goal is to keep that muscle in spasm because the spasm works as a protective measure. It is called "protective muscle spasm reflex." And as long as the spastic muscle sends alpha signals, the nervous system will continue to send its gamma signals back; on and on it goes. This is why a spasm in a muscle can last for years, and often in a location that is not in the same place as where you feel the symptoms. All the while, the autonomic nervous system may be trying to protect the muscle. This dynamic results in health problems and debilitating pain.

Let me take a moment to be clear that a muscle spasm is not a medical condition. It is a physical condition of the body and it is being used as a defense mechanism against what might be perceived as a threat to normal activity. The muscle is locked in contraction and has lost its ability to lengthen. And while a muscle spasm may not begin as a medical condition, it can certainly develop into one if left untreated. A spasm can compress many blood vessels. There are about 60,000 blood vessels in the body, which is equivalent to the length of almost 2.5 times around the earth. Muscle spasms compromise blood circulation and slow down the supply of oxygen and nutrients into the muscles. They also prevent the removal of waste products, such as lactic acid, out of the muscles.

Strain Counterstrain Really Works

If you're in the grip of lower back pain right now, you know how tough it is to get the discomfort under control. And now that you know the role of the autonomic nervous system in creating your pain, it's understandable that massage, stretching, and exercising, as you probably tried in the past, will not have much impact on the protective muscle spasm reflex mechanism. Sometimes it might even be counterproductive and exacerbate the spastic condition because these therapeutic modalities will increase the alpha signal activity from the muscle fibers, and keep over-stimulating the autonomic nervous system which keeps the muscle in spasm. So even though you're trying to heal, with each passing day, your frustration increases while your pain remains.

I saw this occur as a practitioner during many years of work in manual therapy, including sport massage, stretching technique (proprioceptive neuro facilitation, muscle energy technique) exercise protocols, myofascial release technique, and joint mobilization. I experienced frustration at my unsuccessful attempts to release a muscle spasm and stop the pain of my suffering patients. But once I was exposed to the Strain Counterstrain technique, something clicked.

It all began many years ago when I first heard about the Strain Counterstrain technique. After reading more about it, the technique made physiological sense. During the training and certification program, I was amazed over and over again how fast my spasms and the other students' spasms were released with such a gentle technique.

To me, the process of releasing a muscle spasm is no different than when we switch on and off a computer. In both cases we manipulate electrical currents. The difference is that in the body these electrical currents are called reflexes. In order to release a muscle that's locked in spasm, you need to break the continuous hyperactivity of these reflexes (electric signals) between muscles and the autonomic nervous system. The Strain Counterstrain technique is specifically designed to accomplish this by switching off the alpha signals (which are signs of distress) from the spastic muscle, so the autonomic nervous system will stop sending the gamma signals (which is the spasm). When the signals stop, the spasm will release. That's because when alpha signals stop, the gamma signals will stop too. As a result, the muscle fibers will release their pressure on blood vessels, improving blood circulation, which means more oxygen and nutrition to the muscle cells, and more efficient removal of waste products, such as lactic acid, out of the muscle. This allows the healing process to begin.

As soon as I included this technique into my practice, my ability to help people increased tremendously. Now, when people come to me in pain—or perhaps they are guarded with their movement out of fear of pain—I can help them.

I first release the spastic muscle and then mobilize the joint which releases pressure and helps it to move more freely with less pain. Once out of pain, my patients can begin to stretch the muscles which are no longer spastic, as well as strengthen the opposing muscles through exercises.

Most often, by the time a patient comes to me, they have already tried all other modalities without success. Maybe they find me through a referral or they find me on the Internet, and want to give Strain Counterstrain a chance. And now, after so many years of applying this technique to my patients, I am still amazed—despite understanding the physiology that explains why it works—at how effective it is at releasing muscle spasm and providing relief.

This technique has been around since 1955 after it was found and developed by a physician named Dr. Jones D.O. He had been treating a young patient with severe lower back pain with the manipulations he had been taught in the school of osteopathy, with not much relief for the patient. The young patient mentioned that he did not have good night sleep, and suggested that he might take a short nap, and then the doctor should try again, maybe with more success. The doctor put him in a comfortable position and the patient fell asleep for 20 minutes. When he woke up, he told Dr. Jones that the lower back pain was gone. It was the comfortable position that slackened the psoas muscle (which was the source of the pain). This outcome motivated him to explore the relationship between the muscle's spasm and the nervous system, and how slackening the spastic muscle and keeping the body in a comfortable position would trigger the autonomic nervous system to stop the protective muscle spasm reflex.

Strain Counterstrain Basics

Even though I treat patients in my Santa Monica practice for different kinds of pain, and many of the maneuvers require an experienced practitioner, there are several releases for lower back pain that can be done effectively at home.

The technique involves putting your body into specific positions that are designed to slacken the muscle that is locked in spasm. Think of it this way: every muscle has two ends that are attached to bones, called the origin and insertion points. By moving these two ends closer to each other, the muscle will relax and shorten, taking the tension off and loosening it. Once the muscle is in this comfortable position, it stops sending the alpha signals to the autonomic nervous system. In turn, the nervous system stops sending back the gamma signals. With the cycle of distress signals interrupted, the muscle is released from the spasm and you can find relief from your pain.

It's important to note that if the iliopsoas muscles stay spastic for long periods of time, they will twist and torque the spine. This increases pressure on the vertebrae, decreases the space between them, and squeezes the disc out of its normal location between the vertebrae. The disc will start to shift to the side, back or front, impinging the nerve root which exits the spine, and cause more symptoms in the form of pain, tingling, and numbness down the legs, sometimes all the way to the feet.

This is the reason we begin to treat lower back pain by first focusing on the front of the body, and not the back where you are feeling the pain. You want to first deal with the cause, and then you can pay attention to the symptomatic area and perform releases for those parts of the body.

The effect of this technique is cumulative. The more you repeat the releases on a daily basis, the more you will provide efficient circulation to your muscles. This makes them less susceptible to spasms and injuries, and expands your safety zone while performing under the demands of the day. So releasing muscle spasms will help not only with pain reduction, but also allows your muscles to work together in unison as one coordinated and orchestrated system.

An additional benefit to this technique is that it will produce a whole-body relaxation affect. The Strain Counterstrain technique will change the operational mode of the autonomic nervous system from the sympathetic mode (fight or flight) to the parasympathetic mode (relaxation). And it will relax you so much that you may fall asleep. This is beneficial for the healing process when you are in pain.

Step-by Step Guide

It's time to alleviate your pain.

Plan to spend 30 minutes a day on this program. Learn one position at a time, or not more than two. I want you to feel comfortable with one spasm release position to execute before you move to the next. There are 10 positions for relieving lower back pain, and they should be done according to the order they appear in this book. It's important to always begin this lower back pain relief program with the release for the psoas muscle. You may be tempted to skip ahead, because it's a natural tendency to focus on the releases that relate to the areas where you feel the worst symptoms. But this is not wise. You must always start with the psoas because once this muscle is in spasm, a chain reaction occurs. First, it can pull the spine, causing it to twist. This usually begins with the right side of the body, because most people are right-handed and therefore more dominant on the right side of the body. Additionally, most people drive automatic cars and end up using the right leg more than the left. The psoas muscle will eventually get tired, and once the right psoas is in spasm, the left will become spastic too.

Next, a spastic psoas can compress the sacroiliac joint, which is the joint in the pelvis between the sacrum (the tail bone) and the ilium (the hip bone), and then compress the thigh bone right into the hip socket. And once this chain of events begins to refer pain to the lower back and hip, the next issue is with the spinal muscles (which are on either side of the spine starting at the sacrum area running all the way up to the back of the neck) that begin to spasm as well.

That's why when you feel lower back pain, it is often caused by disturbances that we can source to the pelvic area and the psoas muscles, which are located in the front of the body.

Proper Position

You will lie on the floor or a bed to perform these spasm release positions. For the positions where you have to elevate your legs, use a couch, chair, or foam block . Any object you can rest your legs on without using muscles to stay in the position will work. If you have a foam block to use, you can also do the releases in bed.

As you will see in the instructions for each release, placing your body in the correct position is essential to relieving your back pain and releasing a muscle spasm. In the Strain Counterstrain technique, the way to ensure that your body is in the right position is through the process of locating what are known as "tender points."

The Tender Points

For each muscle that needs to be released, there is a corresponding tender point that relates to a specific muscle, or to the location of the restriction along the spine. Pressing on this tender point is how you will find the point, as well as how you will determine if the spasm has released. These tender points reveal if a muscle is in spasm and if there is a restriction along the spine.

Working with your tender points can be done with your index finger, middle finger, both fingers together, or thumb. It all depends on the position you are in and which finger is more comfortable to use. For example, with the psoas release it is easiest to use the index finger. For the quadratus lumborum release, it's more comfortable to find the tender point with the thumb.

There are two types of pressure you will use with your finger: a deep poke and a light touch. The deep poke will be put to use for three purposes: 1) to first locate the tender point for the release you're performing; 2) to determine if you have placed your body in the correct position for the release; and 3) at the end of a release to check if the release was successful.

Meanwhile, the light touch will be used mostly to maintain the location of the tender point with your finger. Once you have located the point, you do not want to lose it. That said, the more you practice this technique, you might begin to feel a pulse under your finger. This indicates an increase in the blood flow as the muscle spasm is released. It's like a boom, boom, boom. The lighter the touch, the easier it is to feel it.

You don't need to feel it for the release to be successful, but if you do, consider it further confirmation of success.

The Release

There are three steps to a successful release of a muscle spasm. Your primary objective is to ensure that your body is in the correct position for each release.

Remember that this technique is effective and comfortable because you slacken the muscle and interrupt the alpha–gamma messages between the nervous system and the muscular system. If you're not in the right position, the spasm cannot release.

This technique is precise and effective, but subtle. It might take time to learn and to trust your fingers, but the more you practice, the faster you will develop the ability. And once you do, you will own it for life!

Step One: Find the Tender Point

1.   With most positions, begin by lying flat in a neutral position on a floor or bed. Your legs are outstretched and your arms are straight by your side. However, any release that is performed on your stomach should be done on the floor only because the bed would not properly support you.

2.   Place your finger on the part of your body designat-

ed for the tender point associated with the release you are performing.

3. With your finger, deep poke two times. The pressure should be four times harder than a normal poke. If it's tender, then you will feel pain and you have located the tender point for that muscle. A muscle in spasm will be tight and tender and you will feel resistance. When you poke a normal muscle, you will only feel pressure, not discomfort. If you do not feel tenderness, move your finger slightly to the left or right, up or down, and try again with two deep pokes. Continue this until you find the tender point.

Step Two: Get into the Correct Position

1. Keep your finger on the tender point, but change to a light touch.

2. Place your limbs and body in the proper position according to the instructions for each release.

3. With your finger, deep poke two times into the tender point to check if your body is in the right position. If you are in the correct position, it will feel 60–70% softer, less tender or both, than the first time you poked. If it isn't yet 60–70%, then change the position of the body slightly and deep poke two times again. Continue this until the tender point is 60–70% softer, less tender, or both.

Note: The more you poke, the more you excite the nervous system, which can make things worse. Limit yourself to two attempts at getting into the correct position. A good metaphor is to think of it as finding a single seat in a ballpark. Maybe you need to move to the left or right, up or down. It takes some fine-tuning to find the correct position, so rely on your finger to feel for tenderness and resistance. Be patient while you learn this technique.

Step Three: Perform the Release

1. Once you have found the correction position, keep your finger on the tender point with a light touch. Do not poke.

2. Remain in position for 90 seconds. You should be comfortable and keep your body in place.

3. After 90 seconds, check your progress by making two deep pokes on the tender point. If the reduction in tenderness is still at 60–70%, then you are done.

4. Gently return to the neutral position, with legs and arms relaxed.

5. Finally, deep poke the tender point two times to confirm the spasm has released. It should still be at least 60–70% less tender, painful, softer, or both.

Benefits of Strain Counterstrain

As you continue to do the releases each day, you will discover there is a cumulative effect to your healing. As more of the muscle spasms are released, a better supply of blood flows to the muscles, which means more oxygen and nutrition and the better removal of lactic acid. Picture yourself as a farmer who is supposed to keep the irrigation system to their field open. Your blood circulation is the irrigation system to the muscles and a muscle spasm will compromise it.

As you begin to feel better, it's natural to think that you can stop doing the releases and your muscle spasms will not return. But remember that you are still using your muscles all day long against gravity. The pressure of gravity is 3.5 pounds per square inch, which is equivalent to 10 phone books on your head. That's a lot of pressure. So instead of waiting for the pain and muscle spasms to come back, you can use this technique as prevention and maintain good circulation to the muscles. The more you do it, the further you expand your safety zone to be able to perform your daily activities without pain.

Daily maintenance of your body through the performance of these releases is essential. It's like brushing your teeth every morning and night. You keep eating every day, so you continue to brush.

Likewise you also use your muscles every day, and they need to be maintained. Do not wait for your pain symptoms to show up again.

Imagine a pain free life in only 90 seconds!

Psoas

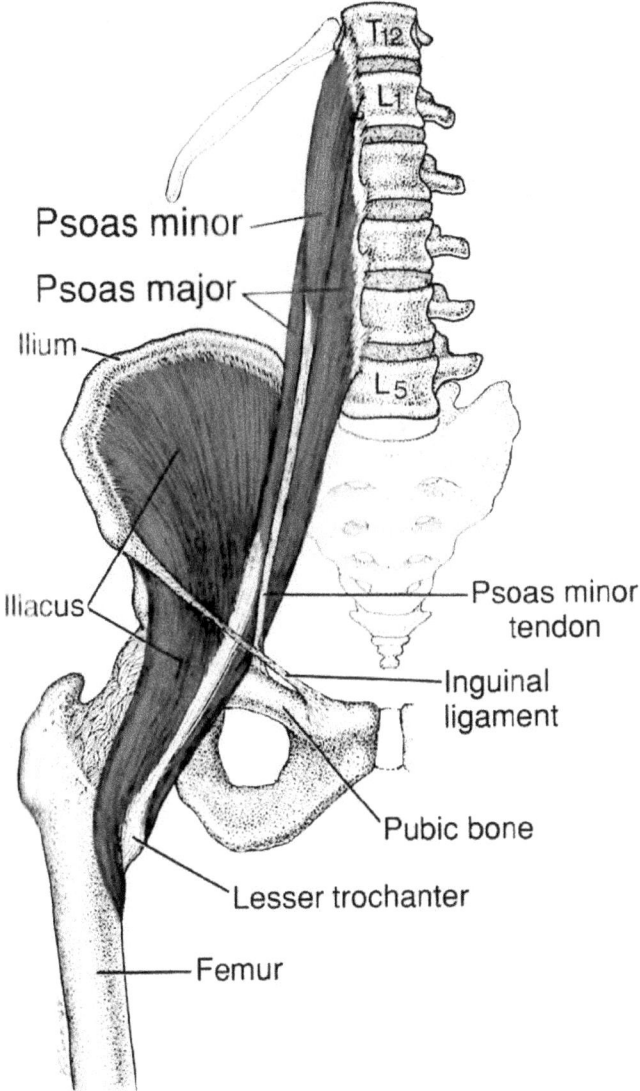

Psoas minor

Psoas major

Ilium

Iliacus

Psoas minor tendon

Inguinal ligament

Pubic bone

Lesser trochanter

Femur

What You Need to Know

The psoas muscle is located on the left and right sides of the lumbar (lower back) area. The psoas muscle connects to the side and front of the spine at T12–L5, passing through the pelvis and attaching at the femur (thigh bone) at the upper leg.

This muscle is the most used and abused in the body, because we use it all the time for walking, standing, and sitting.

Where You Feel the Pain

A spastic psoas muscle usually refers pain to the lower back, on the same side as the spasm.

You can also feel pain in the front of the body, around the location of the muscle itself: in the hip, abdomen, and upper part of the leg.

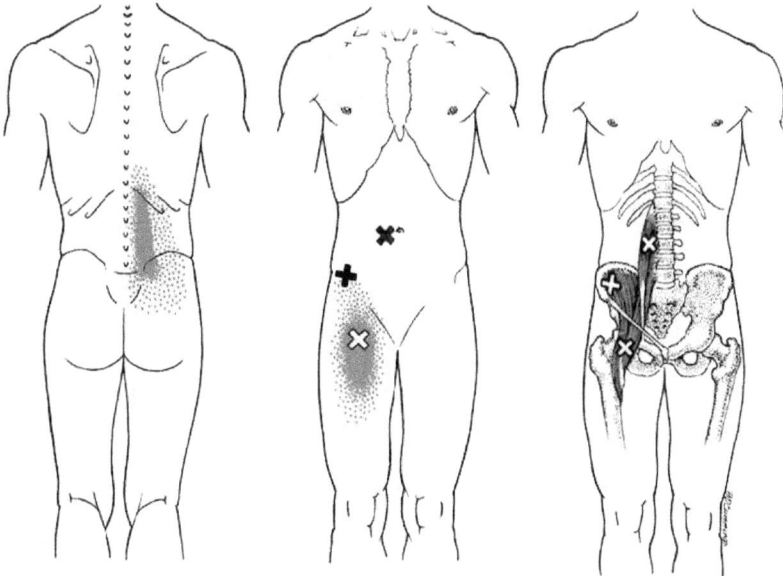

From Travell and Simmons' *Myofascial Pain and Dysfunction: The Trigger Point Manual V. 1 and 2* Copyright © 1998 and 1992 by Wolters Kluwer Brown.

How to Perform the Release

For this release, there are four tender points to locate: two on the right side (one upper, one lower) and two on the left side (one upper and one lower).

Perform this release 4 times, once for each of the 4 tender points (meaning: twice on the right side of the body, and twice on the left side). Be sure to start with the side of the body where the tender points are most painful. Usually, for most people, this is the right side.

As you perform this release, you may discover that when you work an upper point, it might also release the lower point of the same side of the body because when you release the muscle, you slacken the whole muscle, not just the point. If this happens, it means that the muscle has been released and you can skip doing the release for the lower point.

Perform the release on the side of the body where the tender points feel sensitive—even if you do not have symptoms on that side. Do not confuse the pain you feel with the pain you feel in the tender points. It's the tender point that determines the side of the body on which you will perform the release.

Find the Tender Point: Step 1

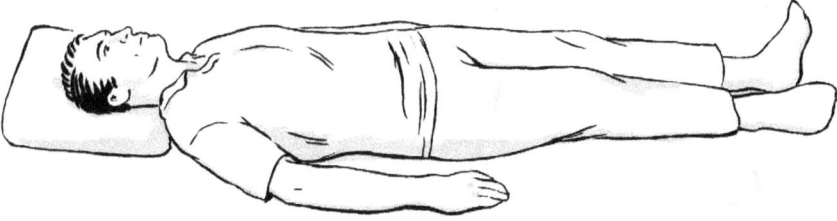

Lie on your back, on the floor or bed, with legs straight and arms extended by your side. You should be relaxed and comfortable.

Find the Tender Point: Step 2

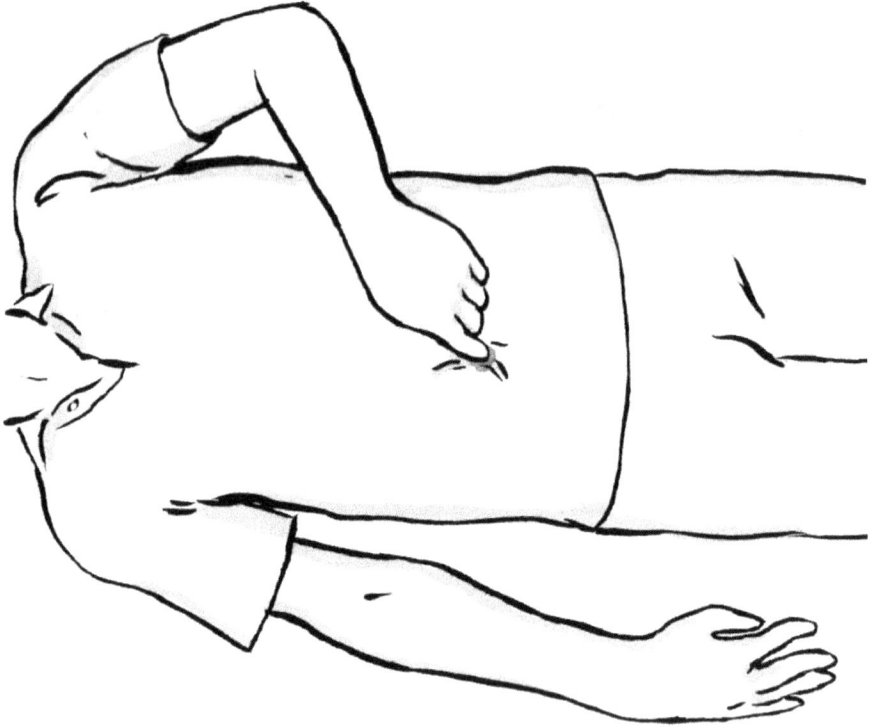

Place finger on the umbilicus (belly button).

Find the Tender Point: Step 3.1

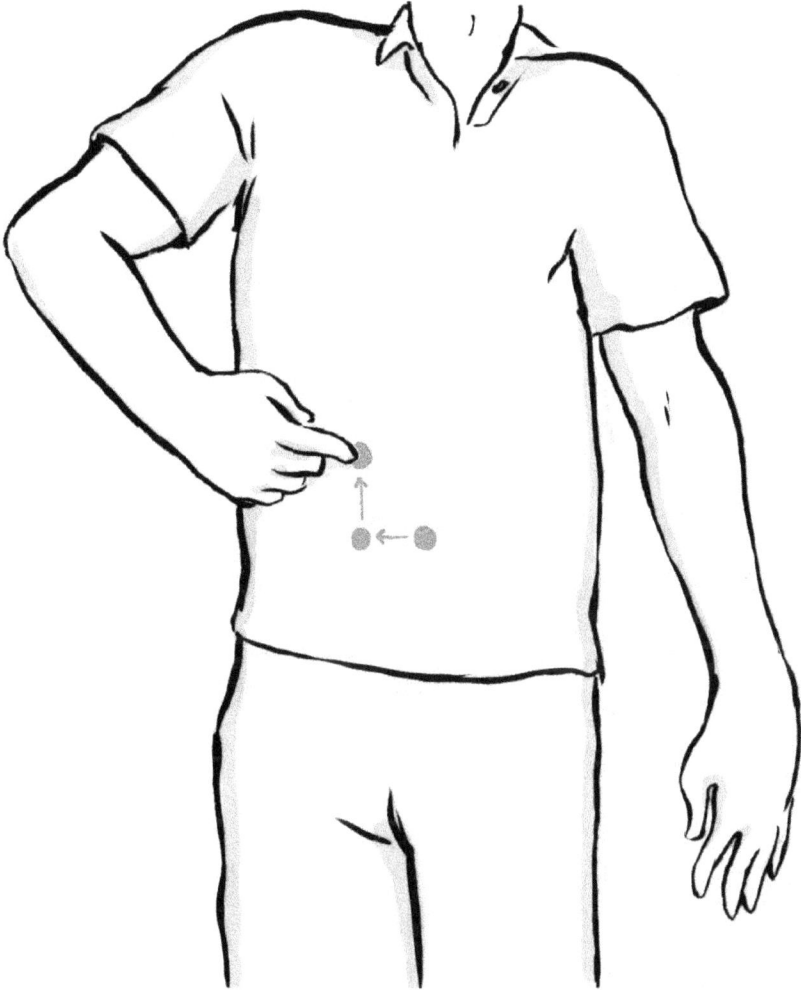

Move your finger 2 inches toward the outside of your body and then 1 inch up, in the direction of your head. This is the upper point. Then from that point, move the finger 2 inches down toward your feet. This is the lower point.

Find the Tender Point: Step 3.2

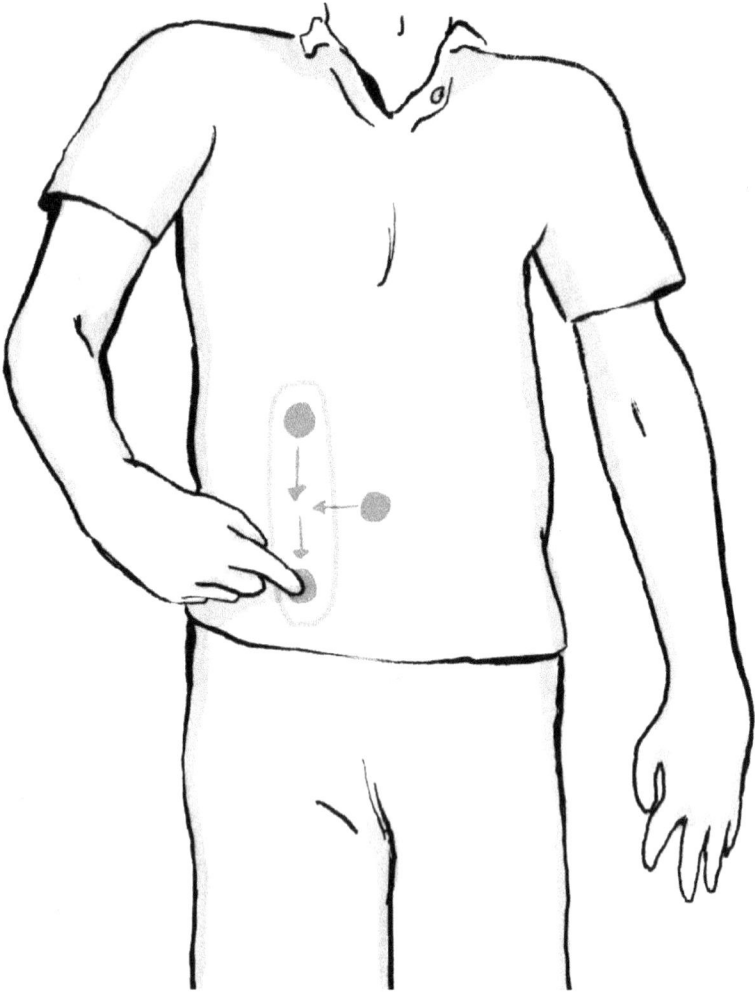

Deep poke 2 times. When you poke, the pressure should be 4 times harder than a light poke because this muscle is deep. It should feel tender, painful, or resistant to the touch. Sometimes, it will feel like a cable.

A tender point is about 1 inch (2½ cm) in diameter under your finger.

Get Into Position: Step 1

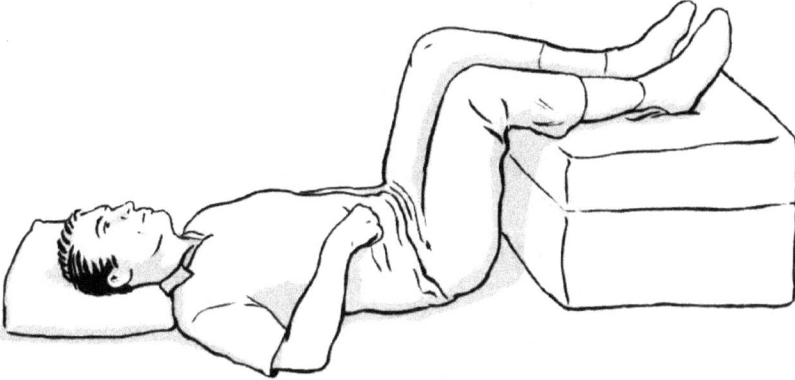

Once you have found the tender point, change finger pressure to a light touch, just to maintain location of the tender point.

One leg at a time, place both legs on the seat of a couch or on a large foam block. Knees are bent at 90–100 degrees. Both the knees and feet are hip-width apart.

Get Into Position: Step 2

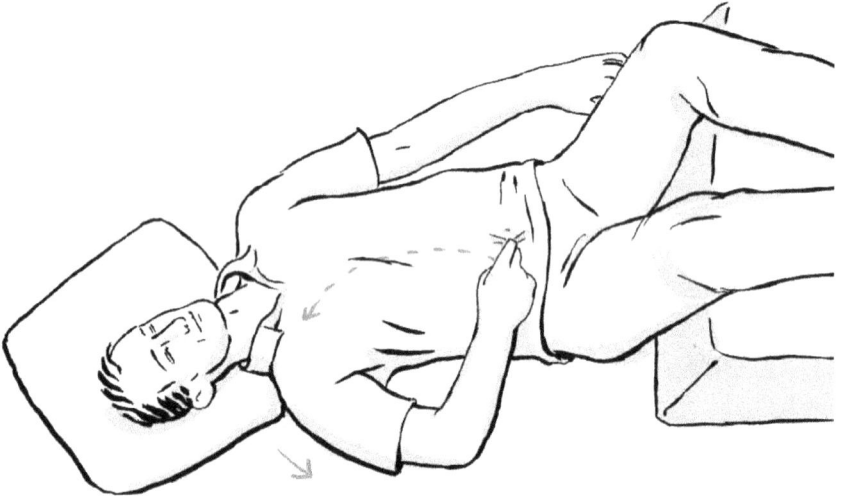

Slide both shoulders slightly toward the tender point on one side of the body, creating a 'C' shape in the upper spine.

Get Into Position: Step 3

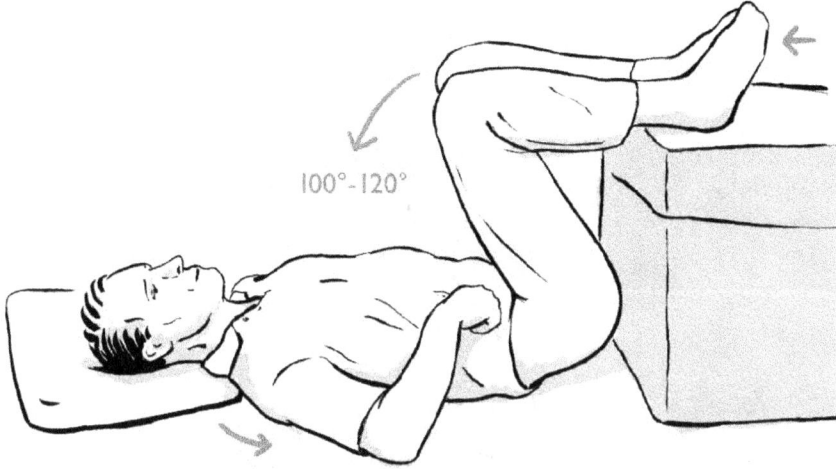

100°-120°

Pull both knees (still hip-width apart) toward your head until they are bent at 100–120 degrees.

Get Into Position: Step 4

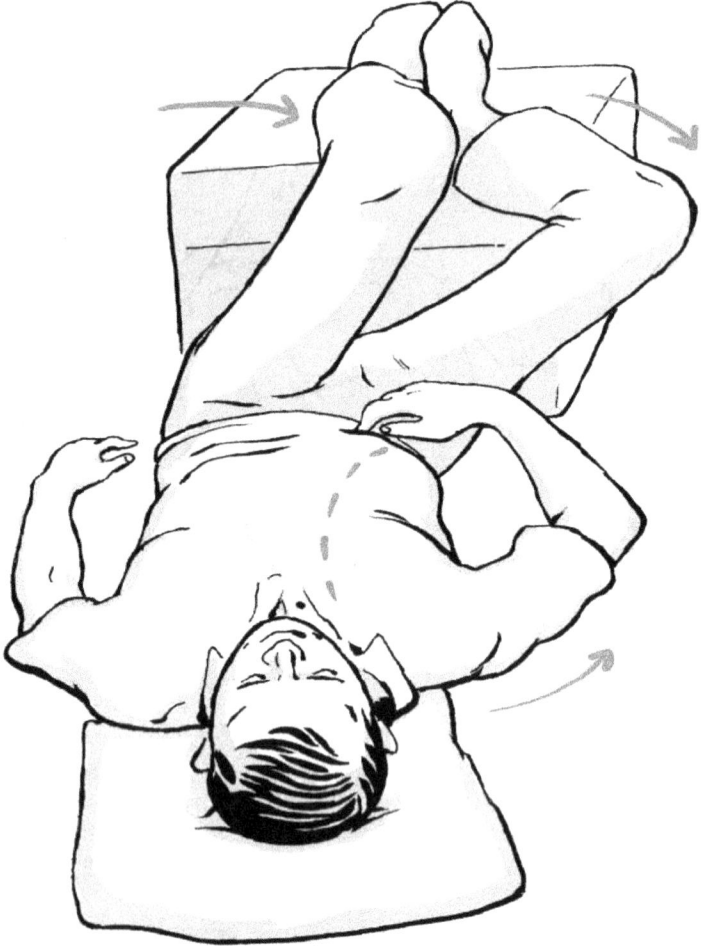

Drop both knees to the side of the tender point, so they are resting one on the other.

Be careful to only flex comfortably. It's okay if there is space between your legs, as long as you are comfortable.

Once your knees have dropped to the side, make sure that the angle of your knees to the floor is 45–60 degrees.

Get Into Position: Step 5

Your body must be in the correct position for the muscle release to take place, so you will now use the tender point to find out if you have placed your body in the correct position.

Make 2 deep pokes in the tender point.

If your body is in the correct position, the tender point will be 60–70% softer, or less tender and painful, or both, than the first time you poked in this spot.

If you are not in the correct position, adjust your body slightly. For example, move your shoulders more to the center or to the side. Next, move your knees higher toward your face, or away from the face; or drop them a little more or a little less. The adjustments are a combination of the shoulders and the knees. This is subtle. Imagine that you are looking for a radio station with a knob. You have to wiggle your body to find the right position for the release to succeed.

After each adjustment, check the tender point again with 1 deep poke.

Continue to adjust your body position until the tender point is 60–70% softer, or less tender and painful, or both, than the first time you poked in this spot.

Perform the Release: Step 1

Once you have found the correct position, change your finger pressure on the point to a light touch.

Hold this touch and your body position for 90 seconds. This is when the muscle release occurs.

Your position should be passive and comfortable with no effort. You must be relaxed and must not use your muscles to hold yourself in place.

Keep your finger on the tender point with a light touch.

Do not move your body. The release is not caused by the pressure of your finger on the tender point. It's the placement of the body which puts the muscle in the correct position so the spasm can stop.

Perform the Release: Step 2

After holding for 90 seconds, make 2 deep pokes into the tender point. It should be 60–70% softer, less tender and painful, or both.

Quality Check

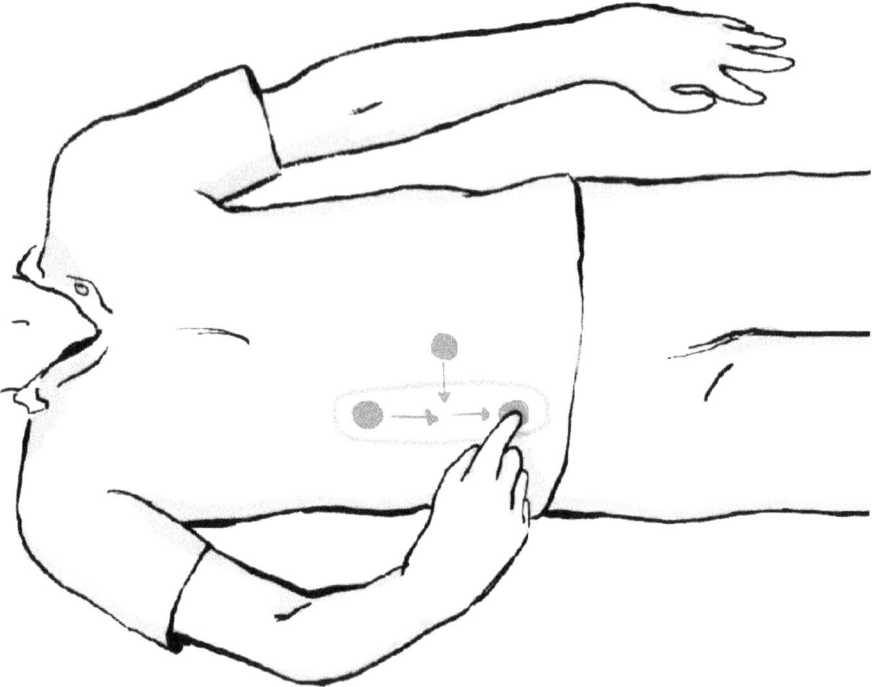

Keep a light touch on the point as you return to neutral position. Move one leg at a time back to the floor or bed, and straighten them. Slide your shoulders back to the center.

Check the tender point one last time with 2 deep pokes to confirm that the release was successfully executed.

This is the real test to determine if the spasm has been released.

Iliacus (center)

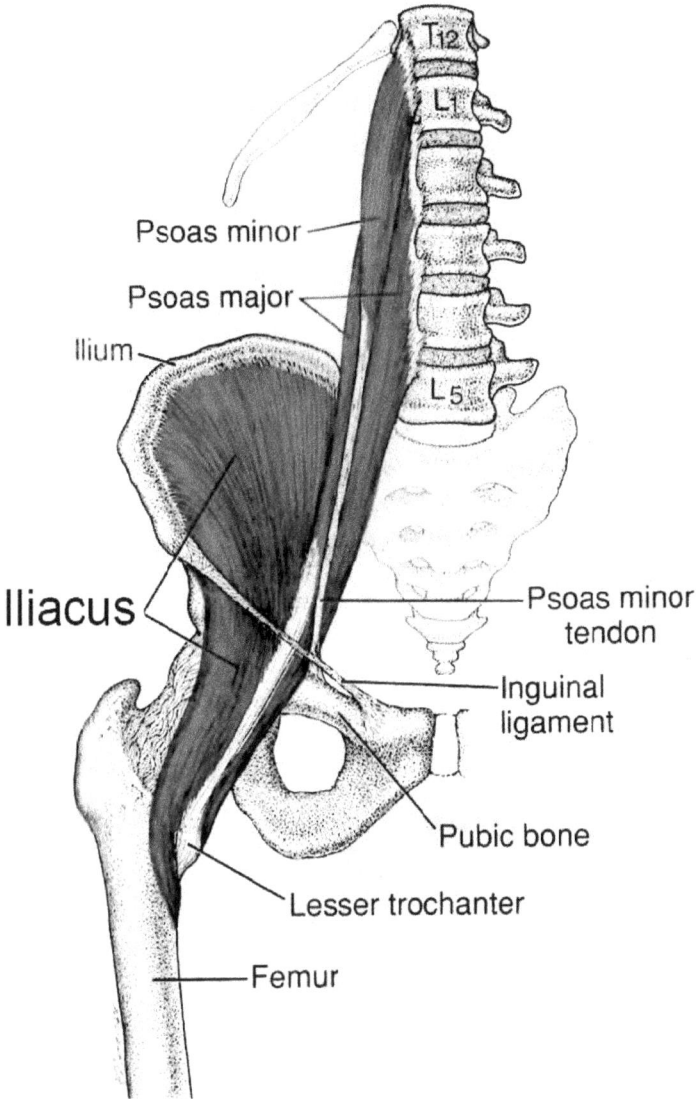

Psoas minor

Psoas major

Ilium

Iliacus

Psoas minor tendon

Inguinal ligament

Pubic bone

Lesser trochanter

Femur

What You Need to Know

The iliacus muscle covers the anterior part of the hipbone, and merges into the psoas muscle into the inner thigh.

The iliacus is one of the muscles we use the most during our daily lives.

It is always used together with the psoas muscle and because of this, the two muscles are essentially thought of as one muscle, called the iliopsoas.

This release focuses on the the center of the muscle.

Where You Feel the Pain

A spastic iliacus muscle usually refers pain to both the front and the back of the body.

In the front of the body, pain is felt on the side of the hip and the groin area and continues down into the upper thigh.

On the back of the body, pain is felt in the lower back area.

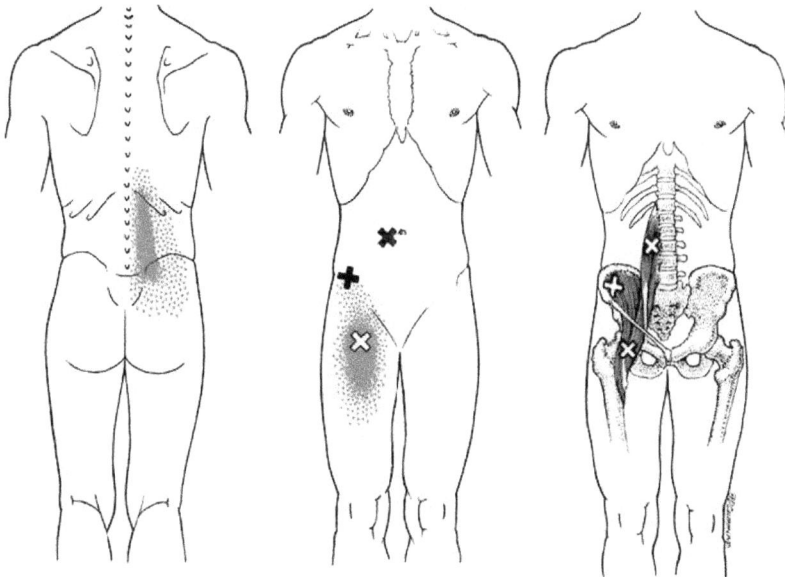

From Travell and Simmons' *Myofascial Pain and Dysfunction: The Trigger Point Manual V. 1 and 2* Copyright © 1998 and 1992 by Wolters Kluwer Brown.

How to Perform the Release

Perform the release for both sides of the body—once for the right side and once for the left side.

Find the Tender Point: Step 1

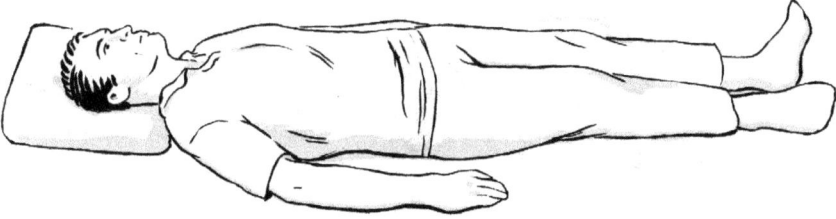

Lie on your back, on the floor, with your legs straight and arms extended by your side. You should be relaxed and comfortable.

Find the Tender Point: Step 2

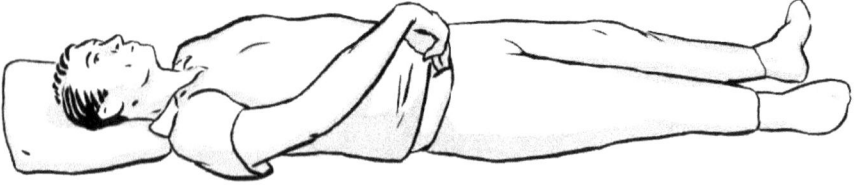

Put 2 fingers together on the front part of the hip bone.

Place fingers on the top of the highest part of the bone; the part that is facing the ceiling.

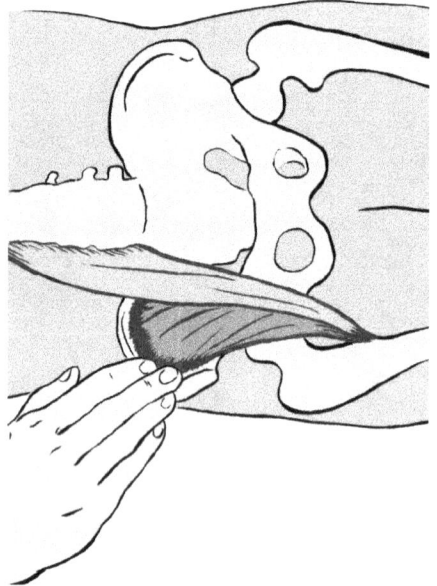

Find the Tender Point: Step 3

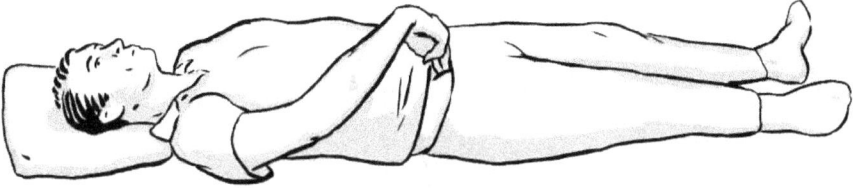

Slide your fingers toward the center of the body, going around the hip bone and into the 'valley' of the bone about 1–2 inches.

The hip bone is like a bowl, so move your finger into the center of the bowl.

To find the tender point, press deep into the muscle by moving your finger down and outward, toward the bone itself. The tender point is inside the hip bone. It is about 1 inch (2½ cm) in diameter.

Deep poke 2 times. When you poke, the pressure should be 4 times harder than a light poke. It should feel tender, painful, or resistant to the touch. Sometimes, it will feel like a cable.

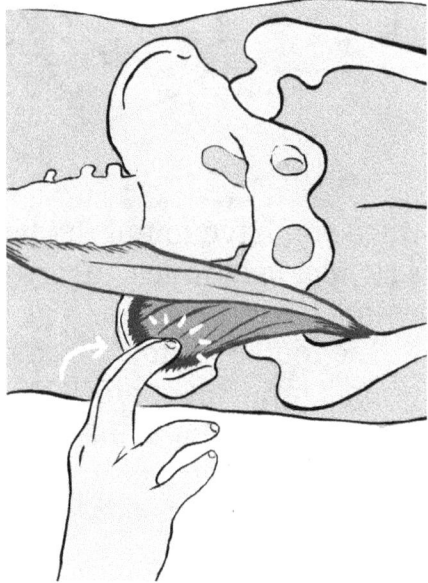

Get Into Position: Step 1

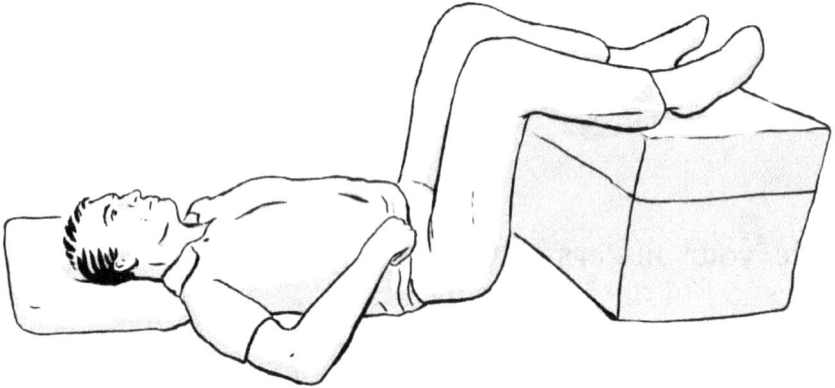

Once you have found the tender point, change finger pressure to a light touch, just to maintain location of the tender point.

One foot at a time, place both feet on the seat of a couch or on a large foam block.

Knees are bent at 90–100 degrees to the floor.

Get Into Position: Step 2

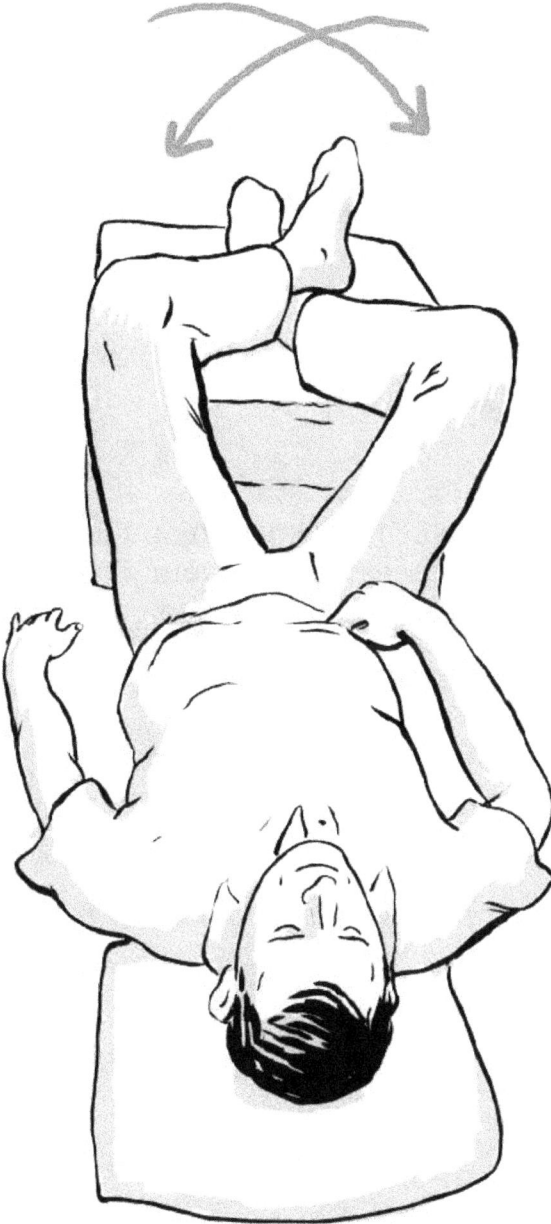

Cross the ankles over each other.

Get Into Position: Step 3

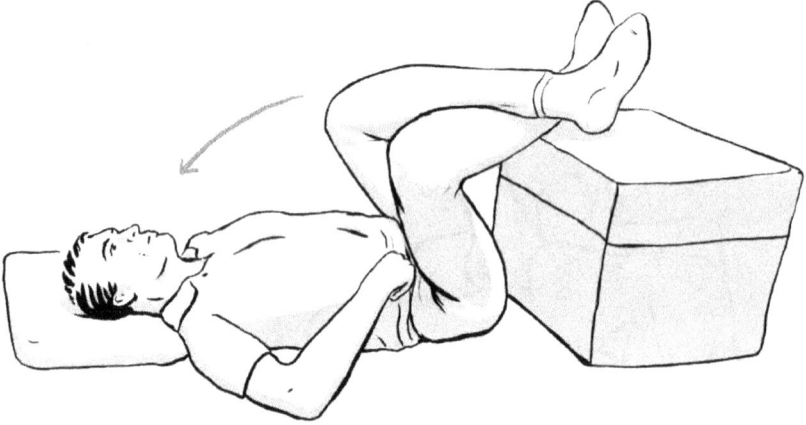

Increase the distance between the knees by pulling them apart. Then bring your knees toward your face to an approximately 120-degree angle from the floor.

Get Into Position: Step 4

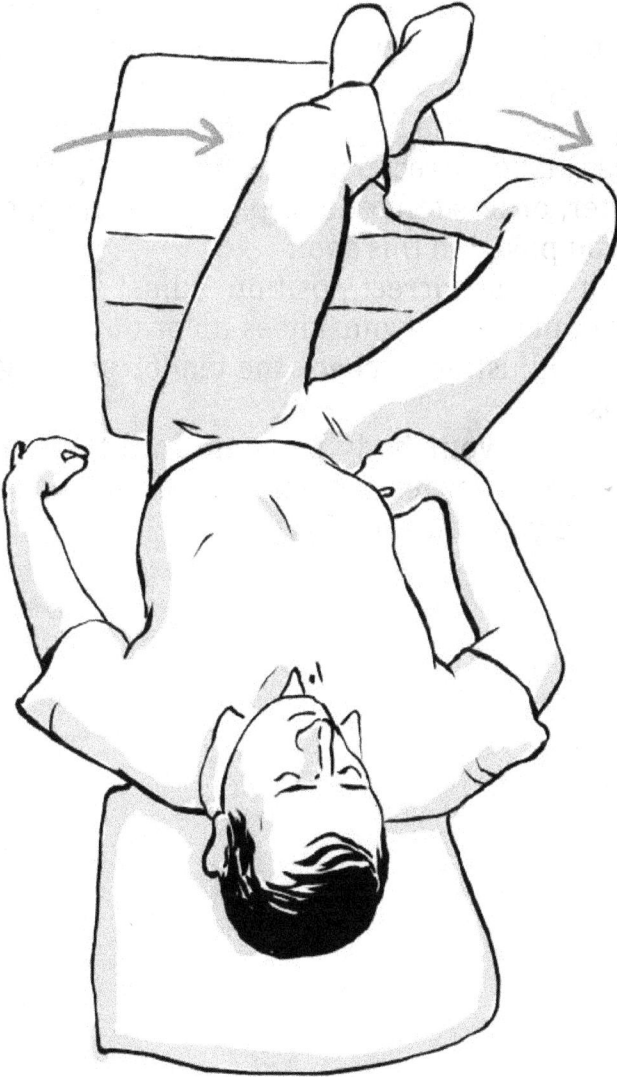

Slide your knees toward the tender point about 45-degrees to the floor. Both knees will drop to the side. They are still separated. Keep ankles crossed.

Get Into Position: Step 5

Your body must be in the correct position for the muscle release to take place, so you will now use the tender point to find out if you have placed your body in the correct position.

Make 2 deep pokes in the tender point.

If your body is in the correct position, the tender point will be 60–70% softer, or less tender and painful, or both, than the first time you poked in this spot.

If you are not in the correct position, adjust your body slightly, for example, move your knees up or down, left or right. After each adjustment, check the tender point again with 1 deep poke.

Continue to adjust your body position until the tender point is 60–70% softer, or less tender and painful, or both, than the first time you poked in this spot.

Perform the Release: Step 1

Once you have found the correct position, change finger pressure to a light touch.

Hold this touch and your body position for 90 seconds.

Perform the Release: Step 2

After holding for 90 seconds, make 2 deep pokes into the tender point. It should be 60–70% softer, less tender and painful, or both.

Quality Check

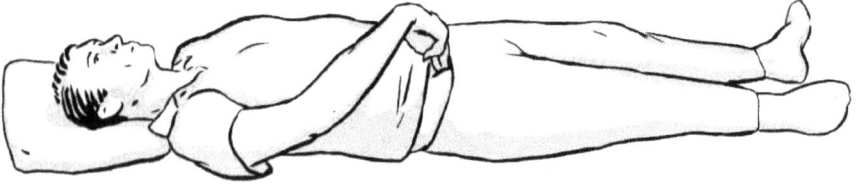

Keep a light touch on the point as you return to neutral position. Move one leg at a time, back to the floor, or bed, and straighten them.

Check the tender point one last time with 2 deep pokes (not more than that) to confirm that the release was successfully executed. It should still be at least 60–70% softer, or less tender and painful or both.

This is the real test to determine if the spasm has been released.

Rectus Abdominus

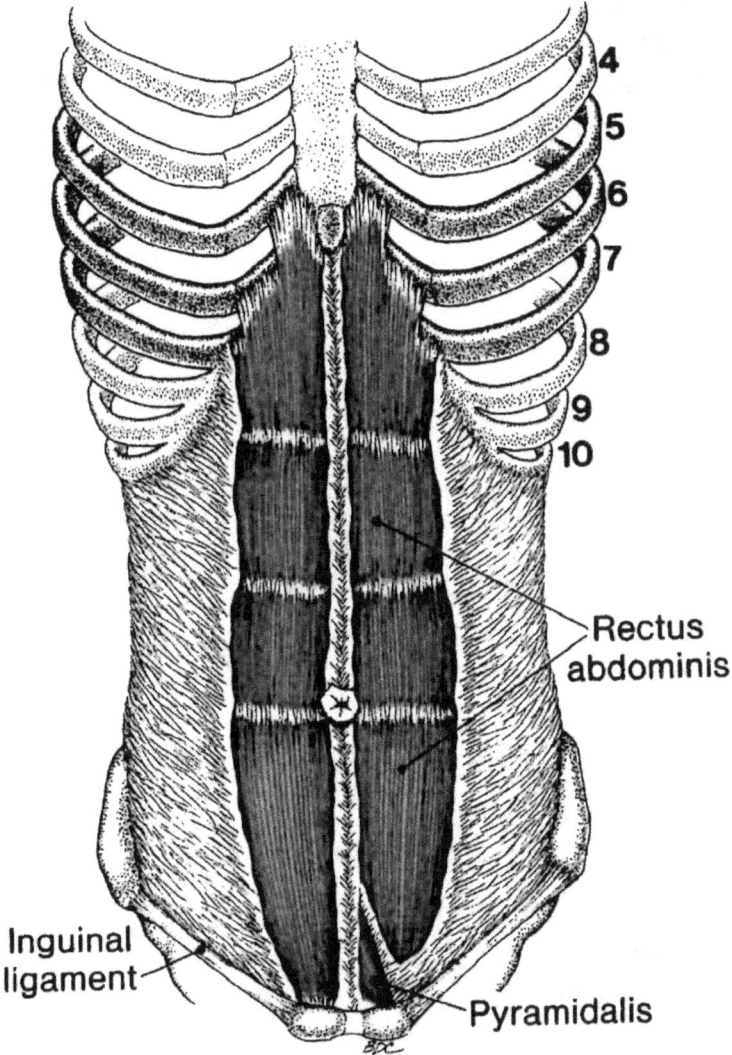

4
5
6
7
8
9
10

Rectus abdominis

Inguinal ligament

Pyramidalis

What You Need to Know

The rectus abdominis muscle is connected from the sternum and the cartiledge of ribs 5–7 to the pubic bone in the front of the body.

A spasm in this muscle can create a restriction in the lumbar 5 vertebrae (L5) in the posterior side of the vertebrae.

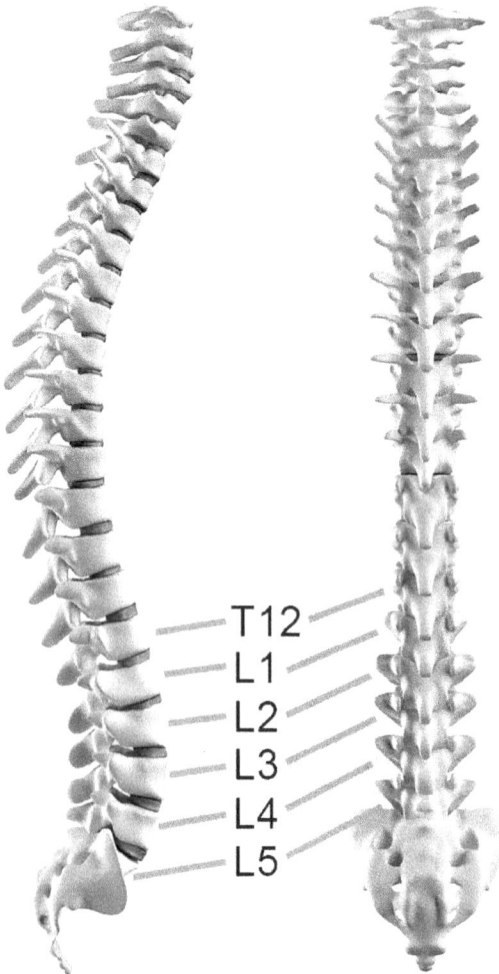

T12
L1
L2
L3
L4
L5

Where You Feel the Pain

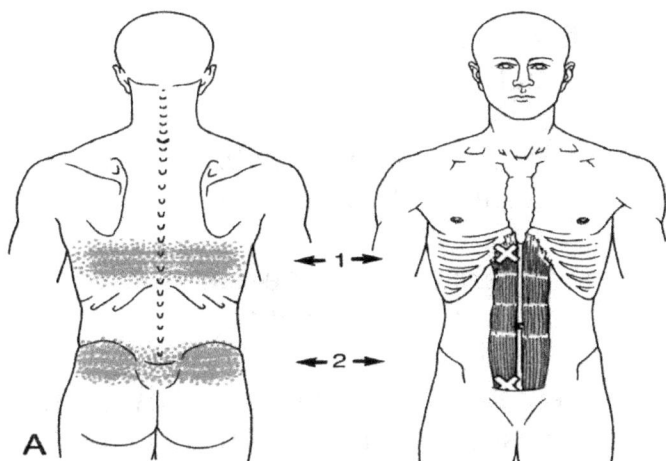

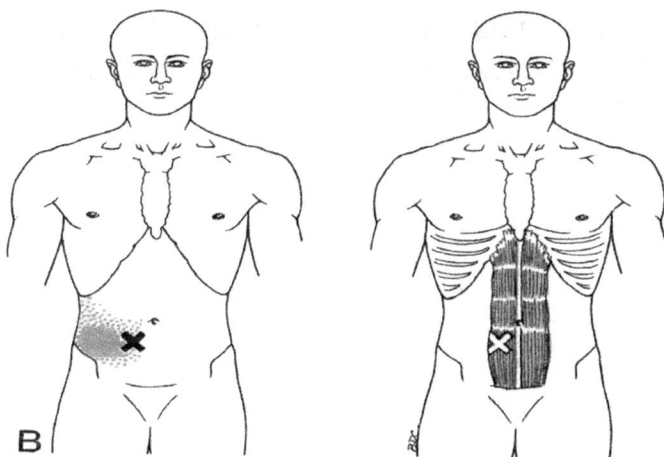

From Travell and Simmons' *Myofascial Pain and Dysfunction: The Trigger Point Manual V. 1 and 2* Copyright © 1998 and 1992 by Wolters Kluwer Brown.

A spasm in the rectus abdominus and a restriction in the L5 vertebrae usually refer pain to the tail bone and the lower back.

You might also feel pain in the knee, on the side of the body where you feel a painful tender point.

How to Perform the Release

It's important to first locate the tender points to find out if they are painful or not.

If the tender points are painful, then you should do this release. If the tender points are not painful, then you do not need to do the release, even if you feel pain in the referred pain areas.

It's important to understand that the tender point for this release is in the front of the body, not the back where you feel pain.

Perform the release on the side of the body where the tender points feel sensitive—even if you do not have 'symptoms' on that side. Do not confuse the pain you feel in those areas with the pain you feel in the tender points. It's the tender point that determines the side of the body on which you will perform the release.

Find the Tender Point: Step 1

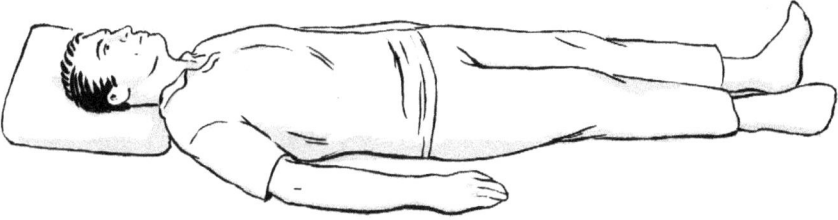

Lie on your back, on the floor or bed, with legs straight and arms extended by your side. You should be relaxed and comfortable.

Find the Tender Point: Step 2

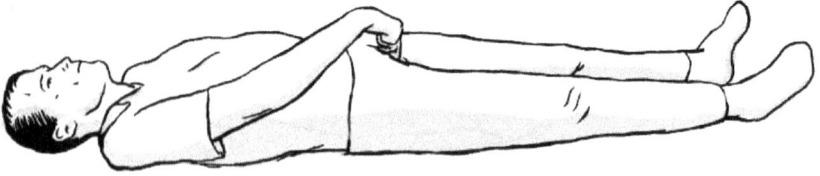

Put 1 finger on the middle of the pubic bone.

The blue dot in the image (right) indicates the correct location for your finger.

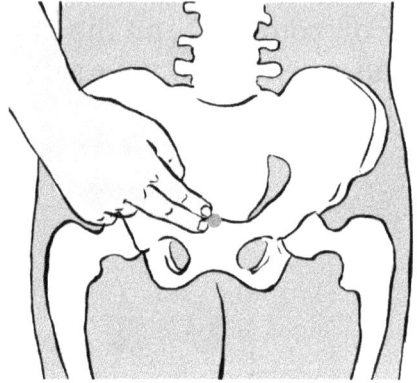

Find the Tender Point: Step 3

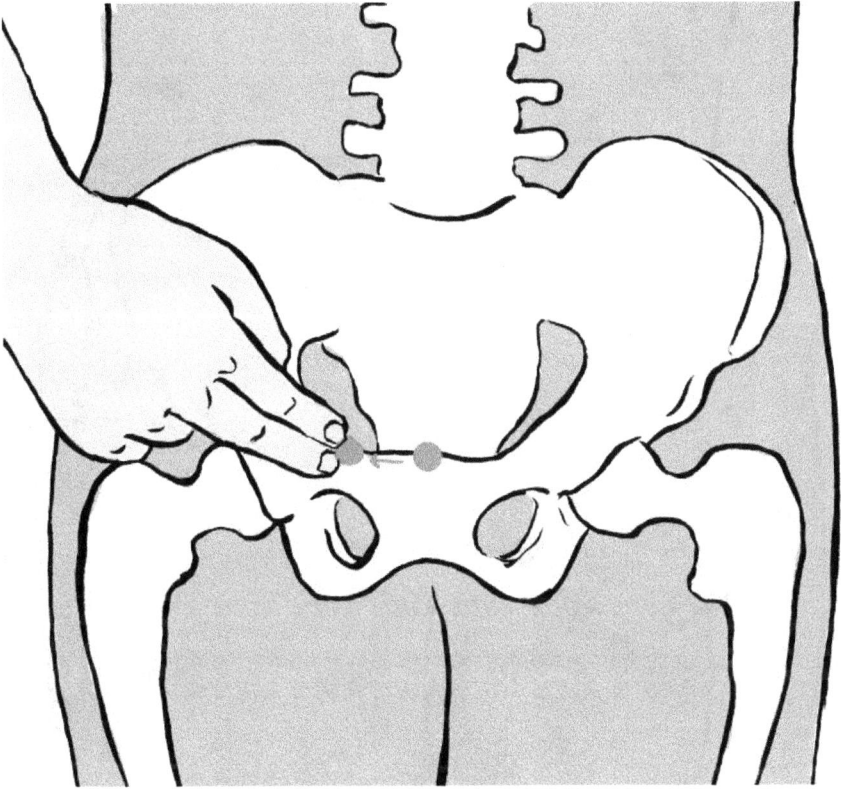

Slide your finger ½–1 inch to the side.

Your finger should be on the top part of the pubic bone that is facing the ceiling.

Find the Tender Point: Step 4

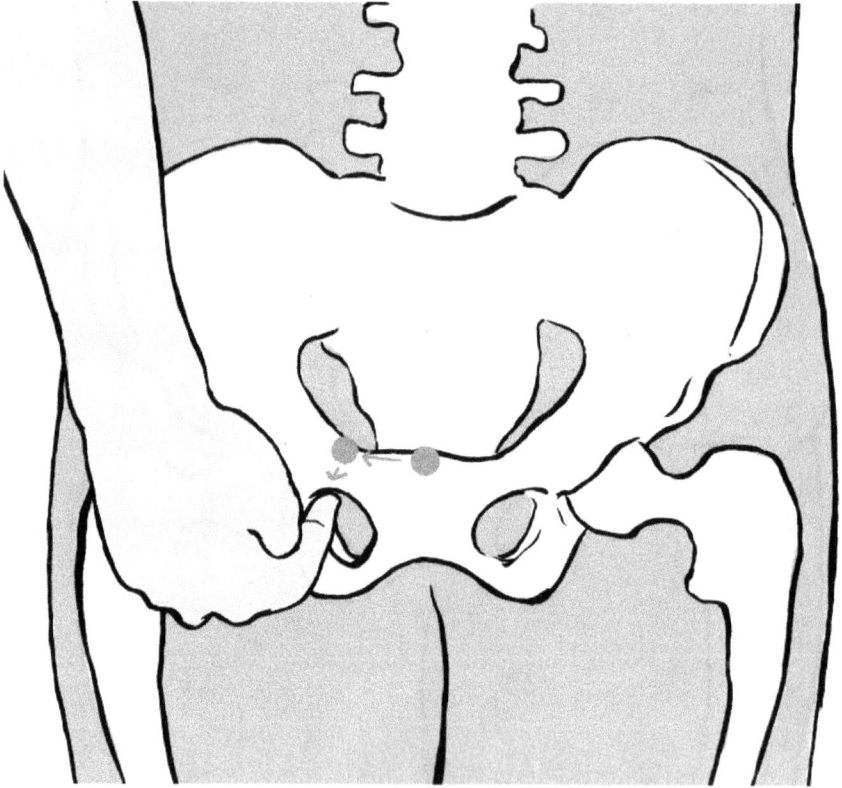

Slide your finger toward your feet and continue over the edge of the pubic bone.

Follow the curve of the bone, until your finger is on the underside.

Now push the finger toward your head.

Deep poke twice. It will feel tender or painful. When you poke, the pressure should be 4 times harder than a light poke.

Get Into Position: Step 1

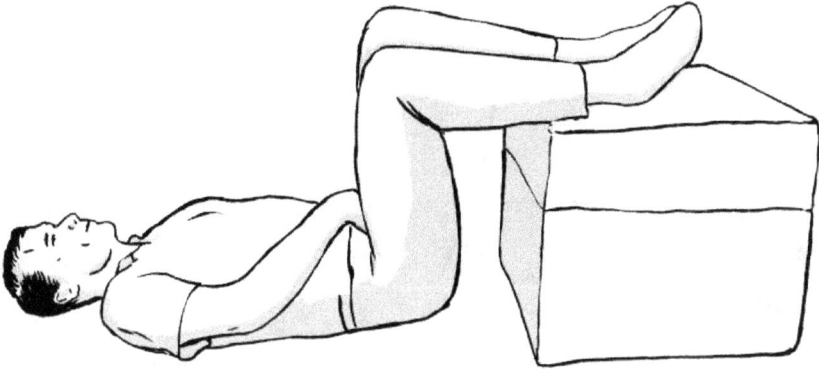

Change finger pressure to a light touch, just to maintain location of the tender point.

One foot at a time, place both feet on the seat of a couch or on a large foam block.

Knees are bent at 90–100 degrees to the floor.

Get Into Position: Step 2

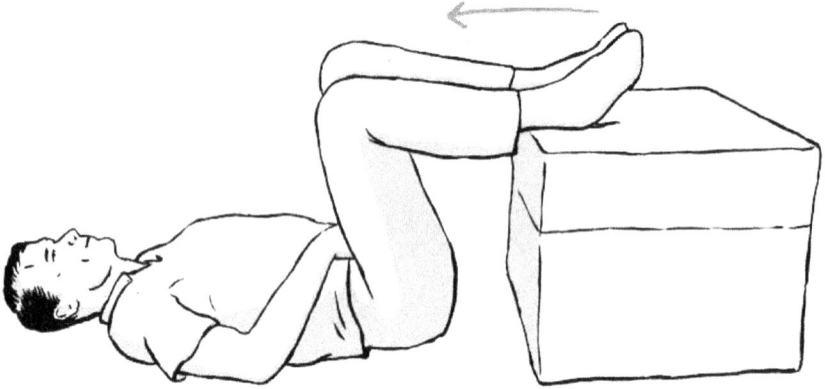

Slowly pull knees toward your head.

Get Into Position: Step 3

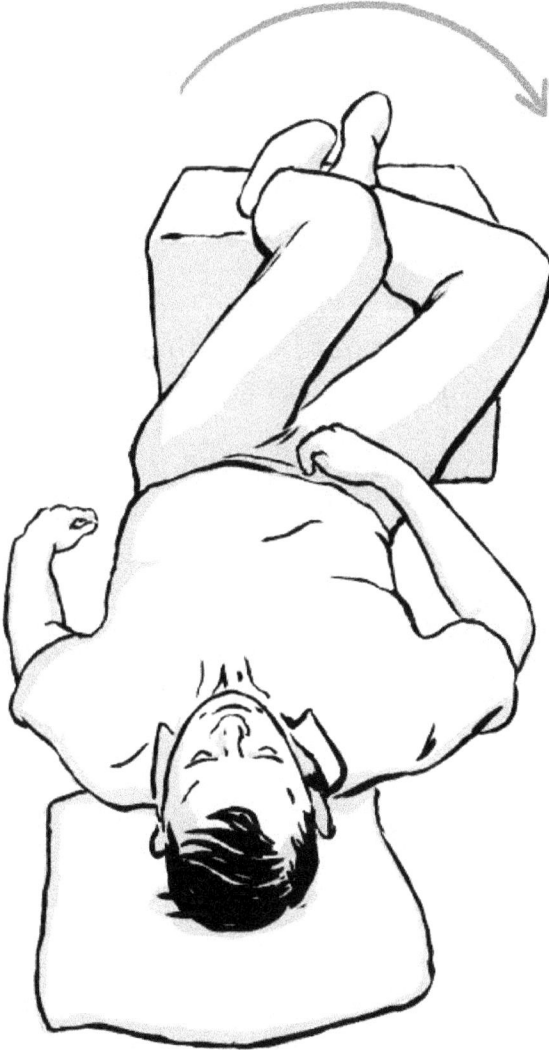

Drop knees slightly to the right if you are working the right-side tender point.

If you are working the left-side tender point, drop knees slightly to the left.

Get Into Position: Step 4

Your body must be in the correct position for the muscle release to take place, so you will now use the tender point to find out if you have placed your body in the correct position.

Make 2 deep pokes in the tender point.

If your body is in the correct position, the tender point will be 60–70% less tender and painful, or both, than the first time you poked in this spot.

If you are not in the correct position, adjust your body slightly. For example, move your knees up or down, or left or right. Then after each adjustment check the tender point with 1 deep poke.

Continue to adjust your body position until the tender point is 60–70% less tender and painful than the first time you poked in this spot.

Perform the Release: Step 1

Once you have found the correct position, change finger pressure to a light touch.

Hold this touch and your body position for 90 seconds.

Perform the Release: Step 2

After holding for 90 seconds, make 2 deep pokes into the tender point.

It should be 60–70% less tender and painful.

Quality Check

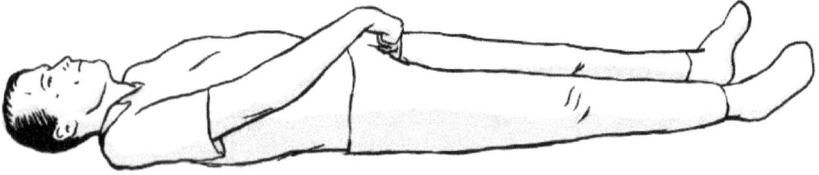

Keep a light touch on the point as you return to neutral position. Move one leg at a time, back to the floor, or bed, and straighten them.

Check the tender point one last time with 2 deep pokes (not more than that) to confirm that the release was successfully executed. It should still be at least 60–70% less tender and painful.

This is the real test to determine if the spasm has been released.

Oblique (lower)

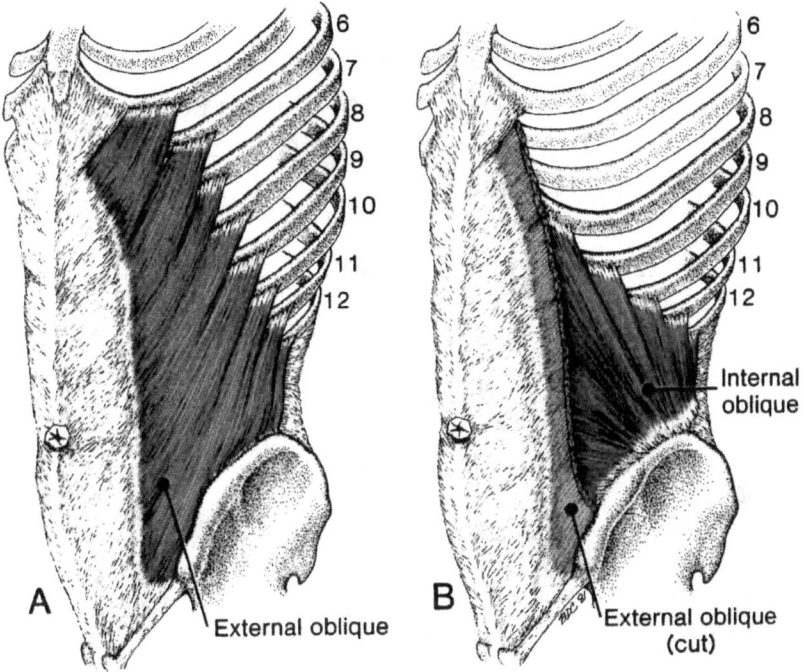

A — External oblique

B — External oblique (cut); Internal oblique

What You Need to Know

The external abdominal oblique muscle is an abdominal muscle in the front of the body.

This muscle is attached above to the outer surface of ribs 5–12, and inserts at the bottom to the hip bone.

When this muscle is in spasm, a restriction can occur in the lumbar 2 vertebrae (L2) in the lower back. A restriction can occur on the posterior side of the vertebrae.

This release focuses on the lower part of the muscle.

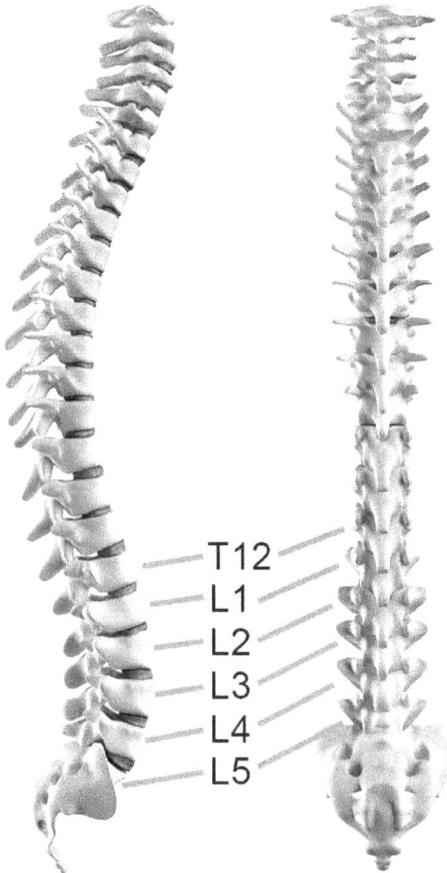

T12
L1
L2
L3
L4
L5

Where You Feel the Pain

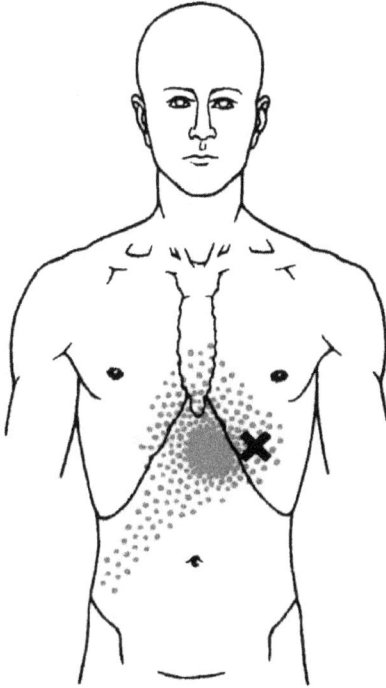

External oblique   **External oblique**

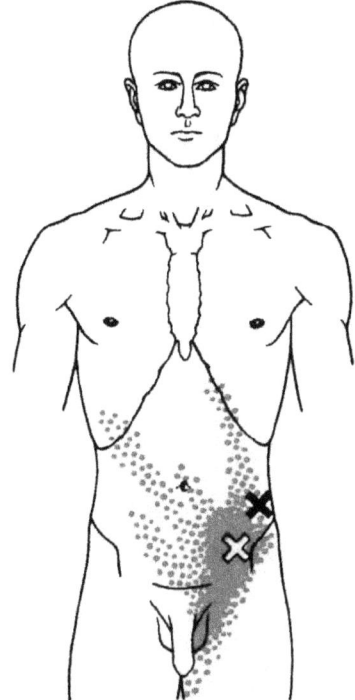

From Travell and Simmons' *Myofascial Pain and Dysfunction: The Trigger Point Manual V. 1 and 2* Copyright © 1998 and 1992 by Wolters Kluwer Brown.

A spasm in the external abdominal oblique muscles and a restriction in the lumbar 2 vertebrae (L2) usually refer pain to the abdominal muscles, lower back, and the front of the hip.

How to Perform the Release

Perform these releases on both sides of the body if the tender point feels sensitive.

The tender points are located in the front of the body.

The tender point for this release is called L2.

Find the Tender Point: Step 1

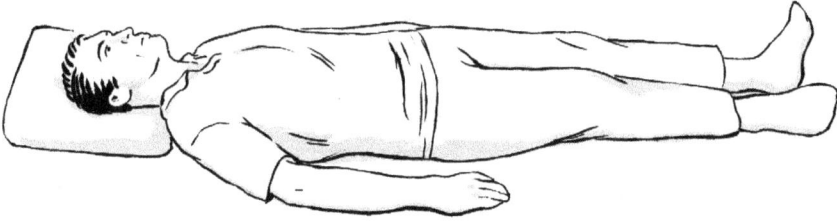

Lie on your back, on the floor, with legs straight and arms extended by your side. You should be relaxed and comfortable.

Find the Tender Point: Step 2

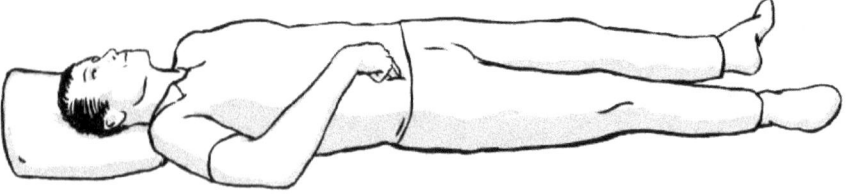

Put 1 finger on the anterior part of the hip bone.

Your finger should be touching the part of the bone that is facing the ceiling.

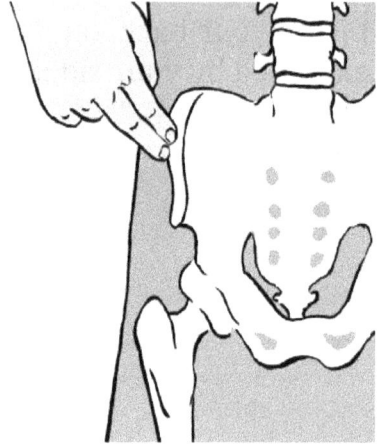

Find the Tender Point: Step 3.1

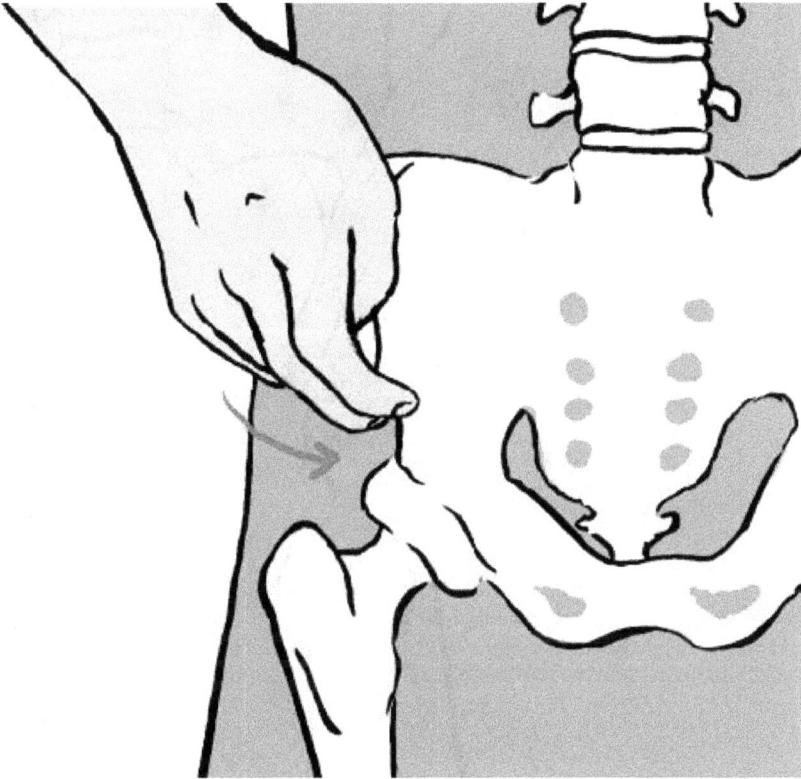

From the top of the bone, slide your finger toward your feet. Slide your finger under the ledge of the bone.

Find the Tender Point: Step 3.2

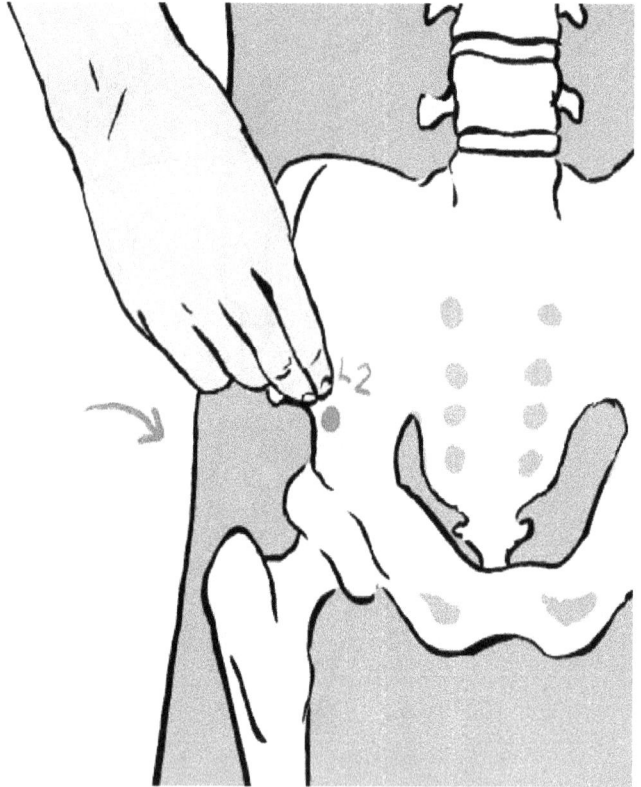

Slide your finger ½–1 inch toward the center of the body.

Your finger will be resting on a tendon. It might feel ropey and tender when you press on it.

This is the L2 tender point.

Get Into Position: Step 1

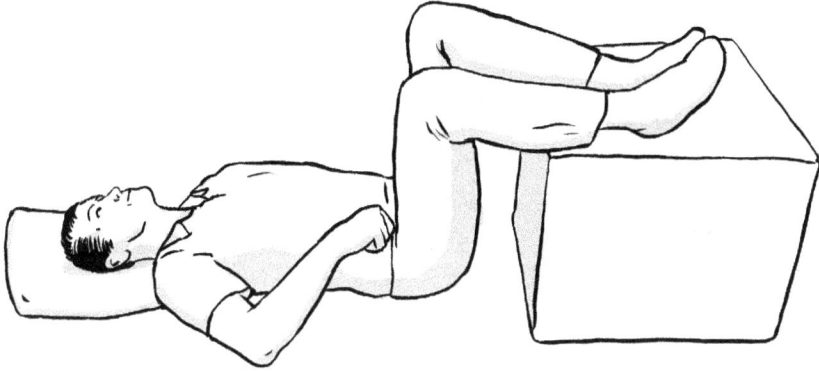

Keep finger pressure to a light touch, just to maintain location of the tender point.

One foot at a time, place both feet on the seat of a couch or on a large foam block.

Knees are bent at 90–100 degrees to the floor.

Get Into Position: Step 2

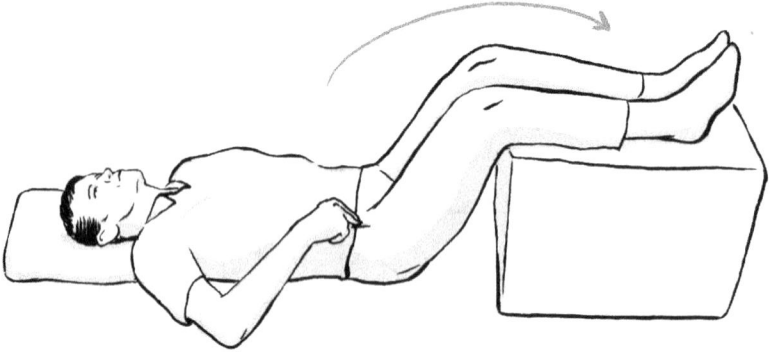

Push your feet and knees forward, away from your face.

In this position, you begin with legs bent at 90-degrees, and as you push forward, stop when the angle is 60–70 degrees.

Get Into Position: Step 3

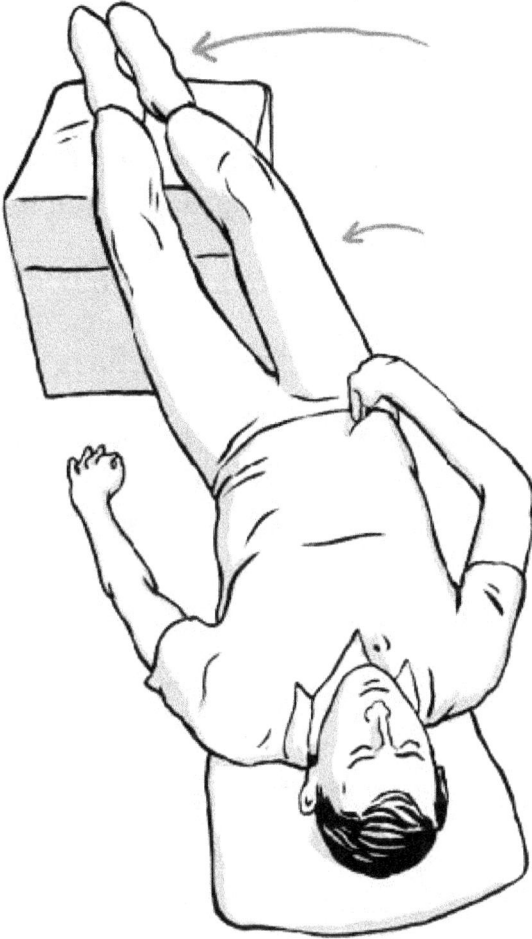

If you are working the right-side tender point, slide knees to the left.

If you're working the left-side tender point, slide knees to the right.

Knees are still around 60–70 degrees.

Get Into Position: Step 4

Your body must be in the correct position for the muscle release to take place, so you will now use the tender point to find out if you have placed your body in the correct position.

Make 2 deep pokes in the tender point.

If your body is in the correct position, the tender point will be 60–70% softer, or less tender and painful, or both, than the first time you poked in this spot.

If you are not in the correct position, adjust your body slightly. For example, move your knees up or down, or left or right, then after each adjustment check the tender point with 1 deep poke.

Continue to adjust your body position until the tender point is 60–70% softer, or less tender and painful, or both, than the first time you poked in this spot.

Perform the Release: Step 1

Once you have found the correct position, change finger pressure to a light touch.

Hold this touch and your body position for 90 seconds.

Perform the Release: Step 2

After holding for 90 seconds, make 2 deep pokes into the tender point.

It should be 60–70% less tender and painful, softer, or both.

Quality Check

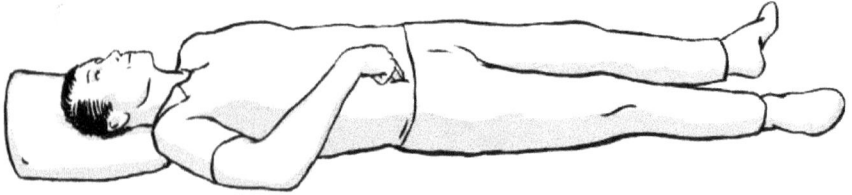

Keep a light touch on the point as you return to neutral position. Move one leg at a time, back to the floor and straighten them.

Check the tender point one last time with 2 deep pokes (not more than that) to confirm that the release was successfully executed. It should still be at least 60–70% less tender and painful, softer, or both.

Iliacus (lower)

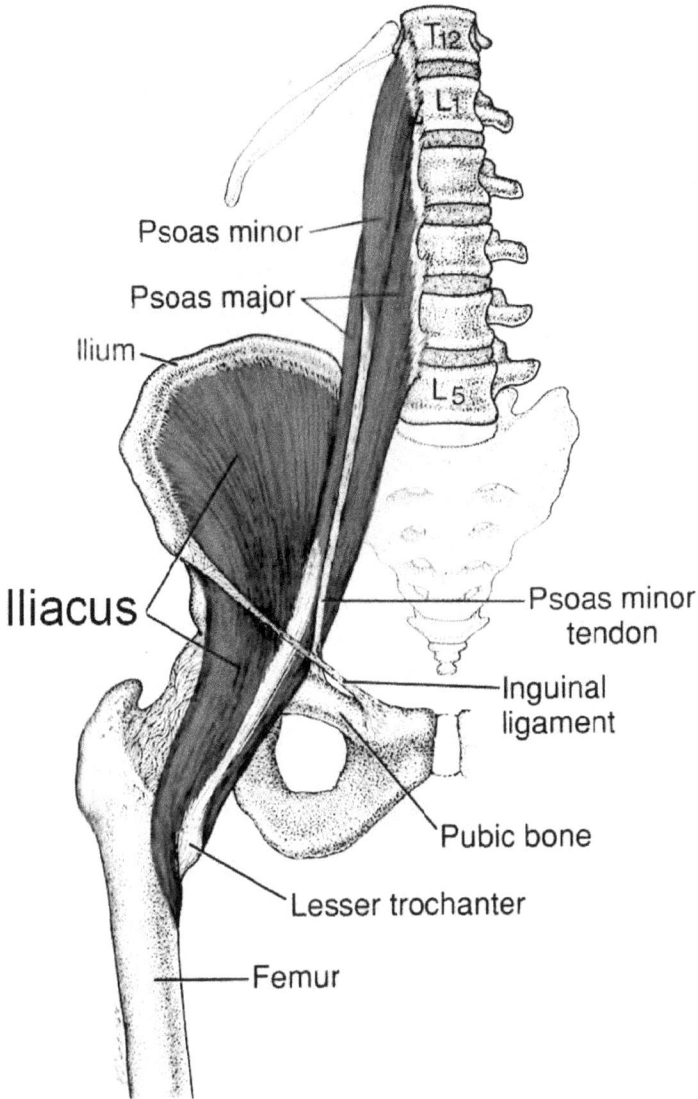

Psoas minor

Psoas major

Ilium

Iliacus

Psoas minor tendon

Inguinal ligament

Pubic bone

Lesser trochanter

Femur

T12

L1

L5

What You Need to Know

The iliacus muscle covers the anterior part of the hip bone and merges into the psoas muscle. Together these muscles insert into the inner thigh.

When the iliacus muscle is in spasm, a restriction can occur in the lumbar 3 vertebrae (L3) and the lumbar 4 vertebrae (L4) in the lower back.

A restriction can occur on the posterior side of the vertebrae.

This release focuses on the lower part of the muscle.

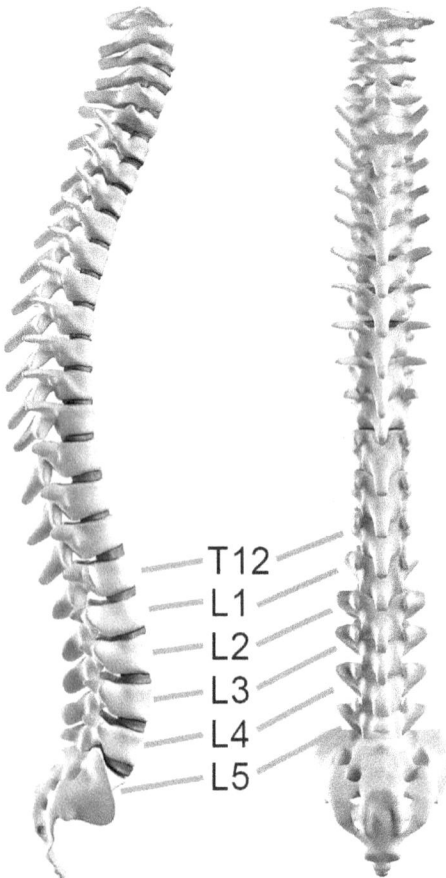

T12
L1
L2
L3
L4
L5

Where You Feel the Pain

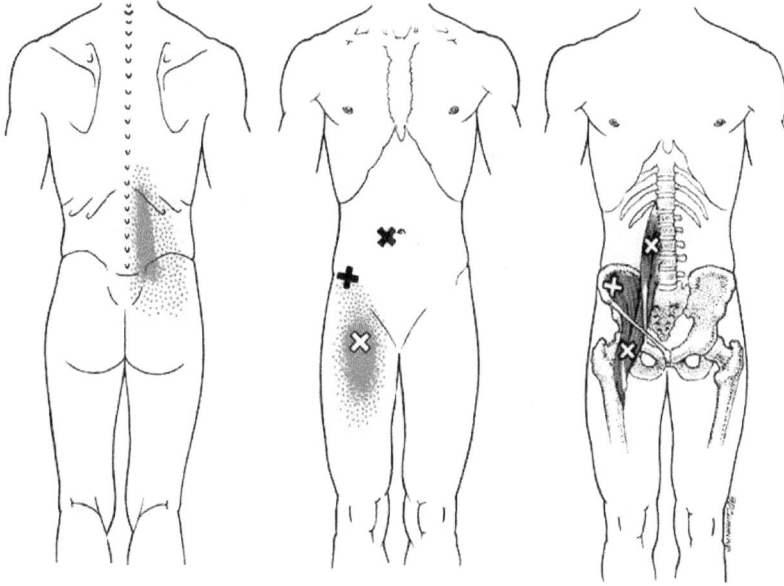

From Travell and Simmons' *Myofascial Pain and Dysfunction: The Trigger Point Manual V. 1 and 2* Copyright © 1998 and 1992 by Wolters Kluwer Brown.

When the iliacus muscle is in spasm and there's a restriction in the L3 and L4 vertebrae, pain is usually referred to the groin, anterior thigh, lower back, and upper pelvis.

How to Perform the Release

For this release, you will be using two different tender points—one is called L3 and the other is called L4. These refer to the two vertebrae that can become restricted when the Iliacus muscle is in spasm.

Locate both tender points of L3 and L4.

Next, perform the release using the L3 tender point.

Then, perform the release using the L4 tender point.

Perform these releases on both sides of the body if the tender points are sensitive.

Find the Tender Point: Step 1

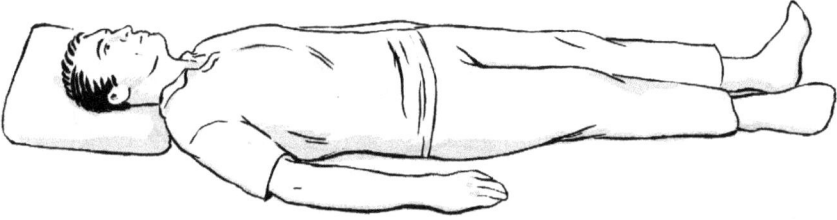

Lie on your back, on the floor, with legs straight and arms extended by your side. You should be relaxed and comfortable.

Find the Tender Point: Step 2

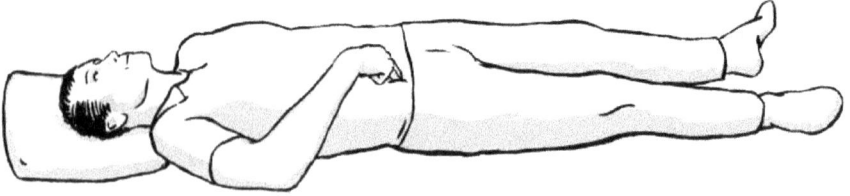

Put one finger on the anterior part of the hip bone.

Your finger should touch
the part of the bone that
faces the ceiling.

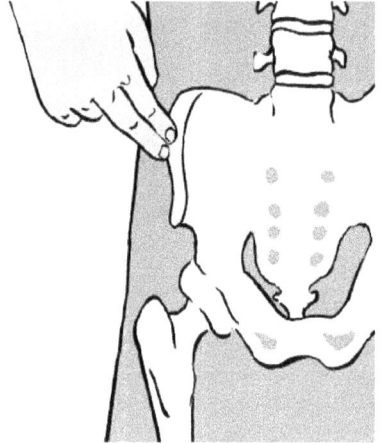

Find the Tender Point: Step 3.1

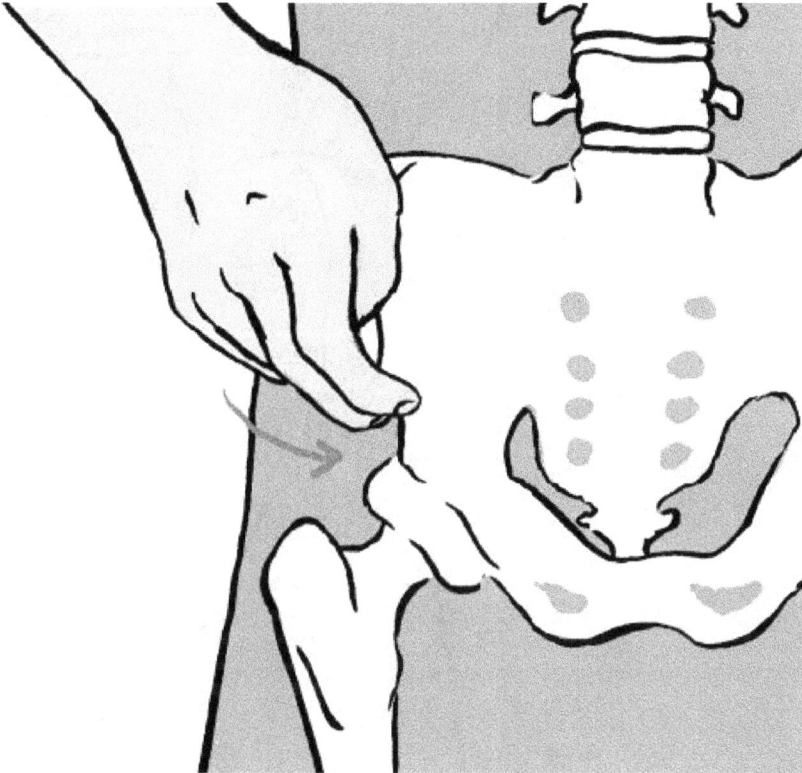

L3 Tender Point

From the top of the bone, slide your finger toward your feet.
Slide your finger under the ledge of the bone.

Find the Tender Point: Step 3.2

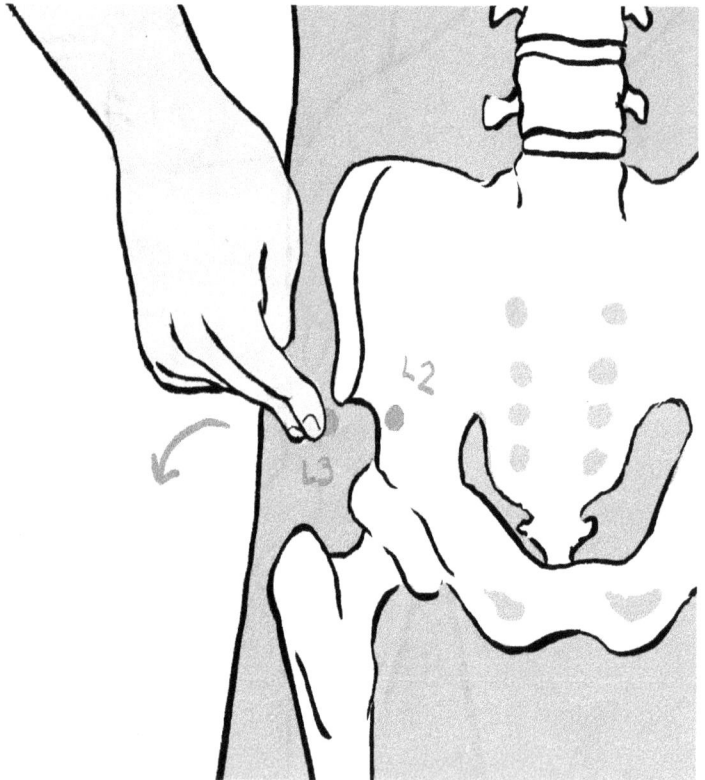

Slide your finger ½–1 inch away from the center of the body.

Your finger will be resting on a tendon. It might feel ropey and tender when you press on it.

This is the L3 tender point.

Find the Tender Point: Step 4.1

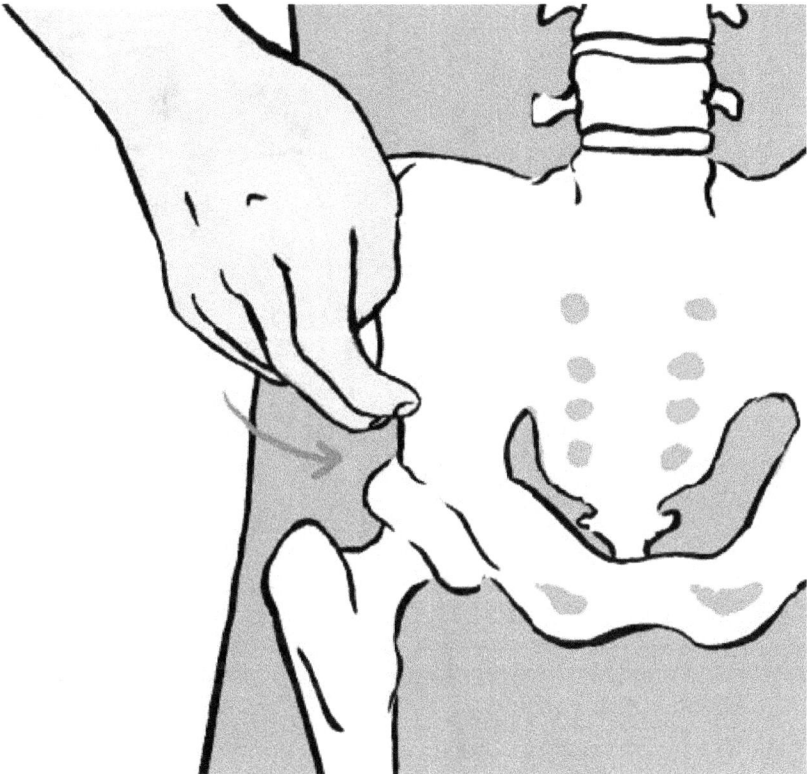

L4 Tender Point

From the top of the bone, slide your finger toward your feet.
Slide your finger under the ledge of the bone.

Find the Tender Point: Step 4.2

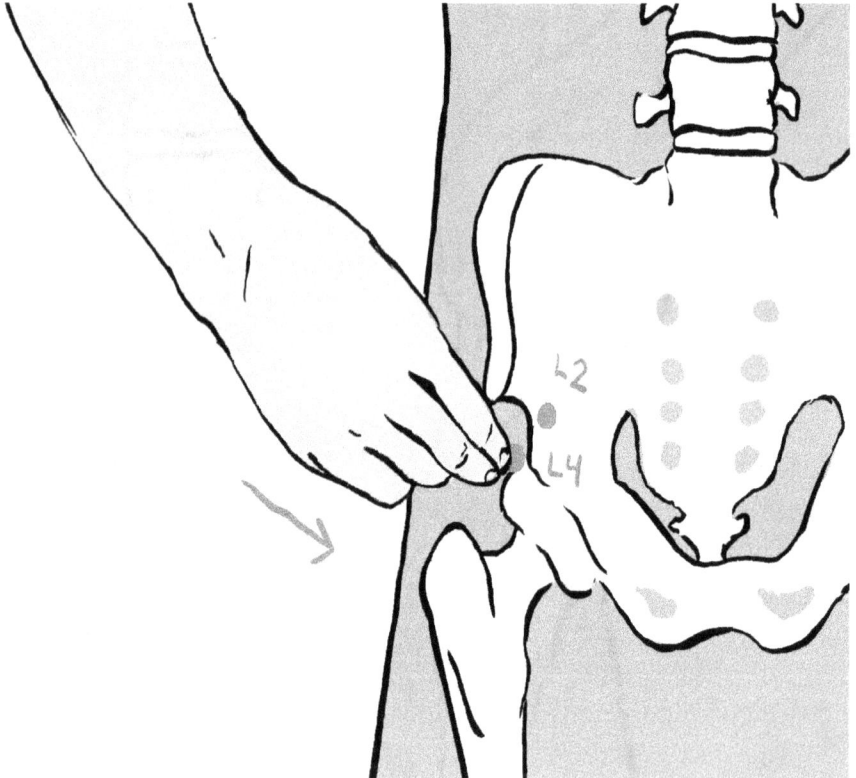

Slide your finger ½–1 inch down toward your feet.

Your finger will be resting on a tendon. It might feel ropey and tender when you press on it.

This is the L4 tender point.

Find the Tender Point: Step 5

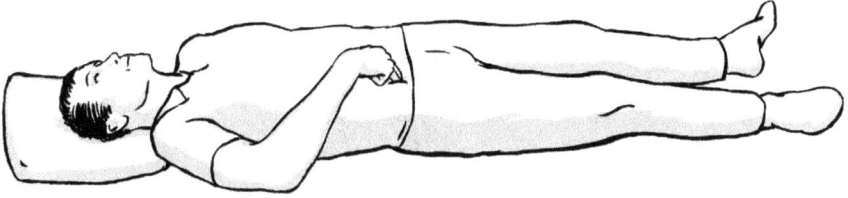

Move your finger from the L4 tender point to the L3 tender point.

Next, you will perform the release for the L3 tender point.

Get Into Position: Step 1

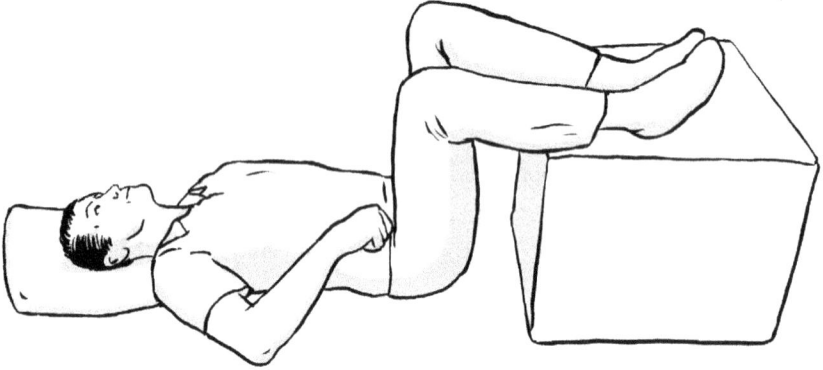

L3 Position

Keep finger pressure to a light touch, just to maintain location of the tender point.

One foot at a time, place both feet on the seat of a couch or on a large foam block.

Knees are bent at 90–100 degrees to the floor.

Get Into Position: Step 2

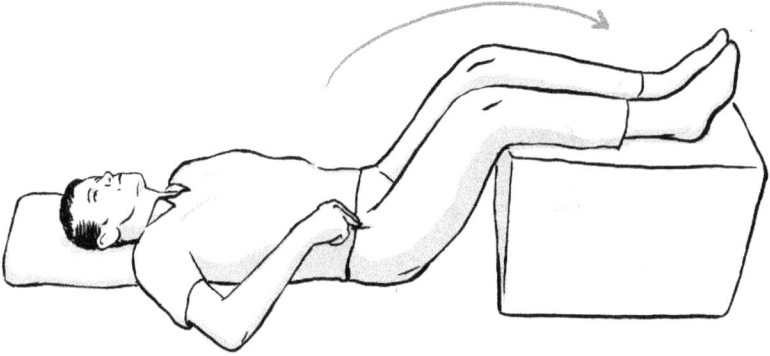

Push your feet and knees forward, away from your face.

In this position, you begin with legs bent at 90 degrees, and as you push forward, stop when the angle is 60–70 degrees.

The positional release of L2, L3, and L4 are similar. The only change is a few millimeters of difference because the location of the points are different. It's the same general position, but you may need to make slight adjustments.

Get Into Position: Step 3

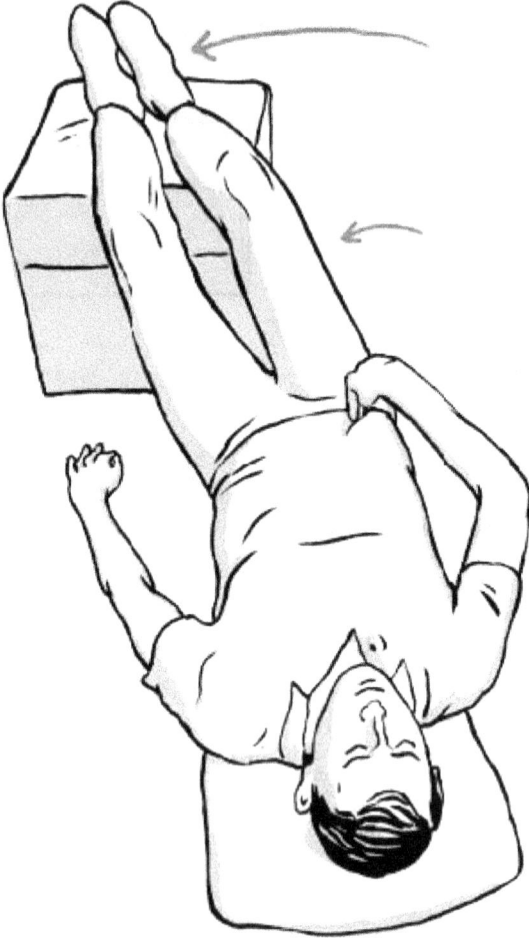

If you are working the right-side tender point, slide your knees to the left.

If you're working the left-side tender point, slide your knees to the right.

Knees are still around 60–70 degrees.

Get Into Position: Step 4

Your body must be in the correct position for the muscle release to take place, so you will now use the L3 tender point to find out if you have placed your body in the correct position.

Make 2 deep pokes in the tender point.

If your body is in the correct position, the tender point will be 60–70% softer, or less tender and painful, or both, than the first time you poked in this spot.

If you are not in the correct position, adjust your body slightly. For example, move your knees up or down, or left or right. Then after each adjustment, check the tender point again with 1 deep poke.

Continue to adjust your body position until the tender point is 60–70% softer, or less tender and painful, or both, than the first time you poked in this spot.

Perform the Release: Step 1

Once you have found the correct position, change finger pressure to a light touch.

Hold your body in position for 90 seconds. This is when the muscle release occurs.

The position should be passive and comfortable with no effort.

You must be relaxed and must not use your muscles to hold yourself in place.

Keep your finger on the tender point with a light touch.

Do not move your body.

The release is not caused by the pressure of your finger on the tender point. It's the placement of the body which puts the muscle in the correct position so the spasm can stop.

Perform the Release: Step 2

After holding for 90 seconds, make 2 deep pokes into the tender point. It should be 60–70% less tender and painful, softer, or both.

Quality Check

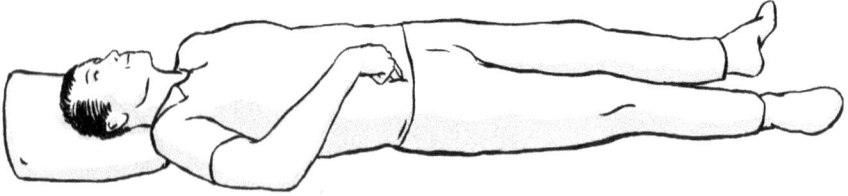

Keep a light touch on the point as you return to neutral position. Move one leg at a time, back to the floor, and straighten
them.

Check the tender point one last time with 2 deep pokes (not
more than that) to confirm that the release was successfully
executed. It should still be at least 60–70% softer, or less
tender and painful or both.

Next, you will return to the first position and perform the
release using the L4 tender point.

Sometimes the release for L2 will release the L4 point.

Get Into Position: Step 1

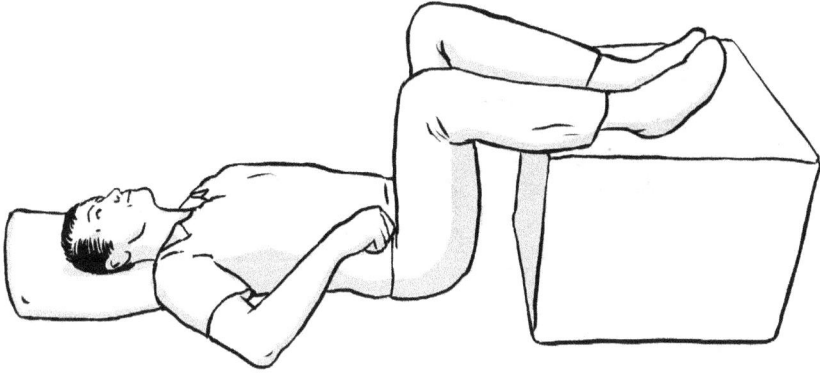

L4 Position

Keep finger pressure to a light touch, just to maintain location of the tender point.

One foot at a time, place both feet on the seat of a couch or on a large foam block.

Knees are bent at 90–100 degrees to the floor.

Get Into Position: Step 2

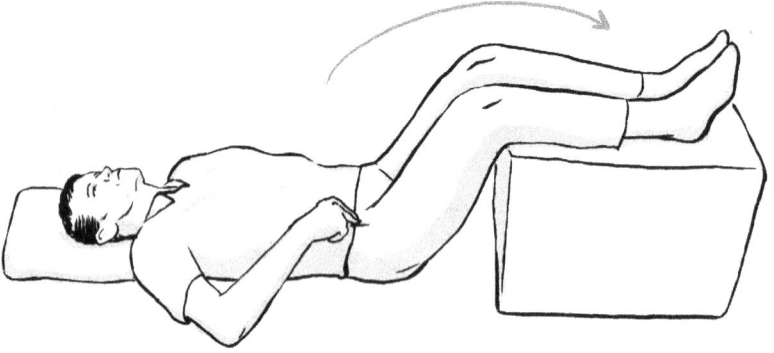

Push your feet and knees forward, away from your face.

In this position, you begin with legs bent at 90 degrees, and as you push forward, stop when the angle is 60–70 degrees.

Get Into Position: Step 3

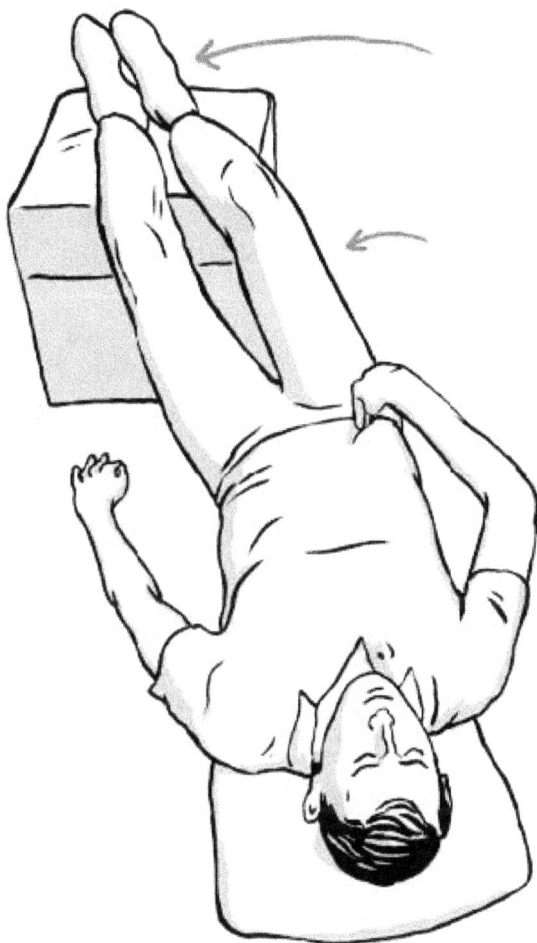

If you are working the right-side tender point, slide your knees to the left.

If you're working the left-side tender point, slide your knees to the right.

Knees are still around 60–70 degrees.

Get Into Position: Step 4

Your body must be in the correct position for the muscle release to take place, so you will now use the L4 tender point to find out if you have placed your body in the correct position.

Make 2 deep pokes in the tender point.

If your body is in the correct position, the tender point will be 60–70% softer, or less tender and painful, or both, than the first time you poked in this spot.

If you are not in the correct position, adjust your body slightly. For example, move your knees up or down, or left or right, then after each adjustment check the tender point with 1 deep poke.

Continue to adjust your body position until the tender point is 60–70% softer, or less tender and painful, or both, than the first time you poked in this spot.

Perform the Release: Step 1

Once you have found the correct position, change finger pressure to a light touch.

Hold this touch and your body position for 90 seconds.

Perform the Release: Step 2

After holding for 90 seconds, make 2 deep pokes into the tender point.

It should be 60–70% less tender and painful, softer or both.

Quality Check

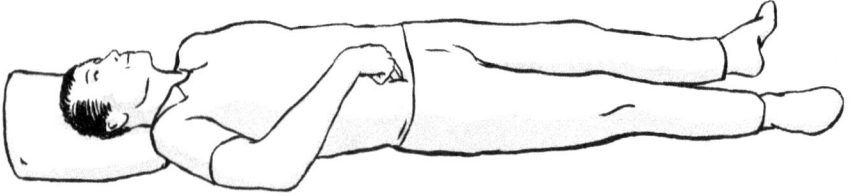

Keep a light touch on the point as you return to neutral position. Move one leg at a time, back to the floor, and straighten them.

Check the L4 tender point one last time to confirm that the release was successfully executed. It should still be at least 70% softer, or less tender and painful or both. This is the real test to determine if the spasm has been released.

Oblique (upper)

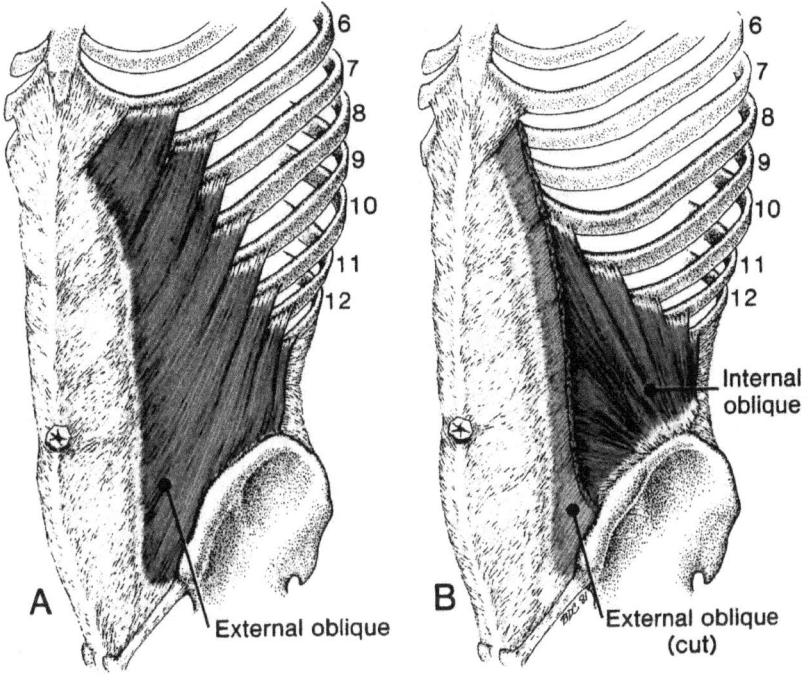

A

External oblique

B

External oblique
(cut)

Internal
oblique

6
7
8
9
10
11
12

6
7
8
9
10
11
12

What You Need to Know

The external and internal abdominal obliques connect the rib cage and the top of the hip into the anterior part of the pelvis.

When these muscles are in spasm, a restriction can occur in the thoracic 12 vertebrae (T12), in the upper lower back.

This muscle might feel painful or ticklish, which is a sign of spasm.

In addition, if the iliopsoas muscle is spastic and weak, the body uses these abdominal oblique muscles (with the help of the quadratus lumborum and spinal muscles) to compensate in its attempt to propel the leg.

This release focuses on the upper part of the muscles.

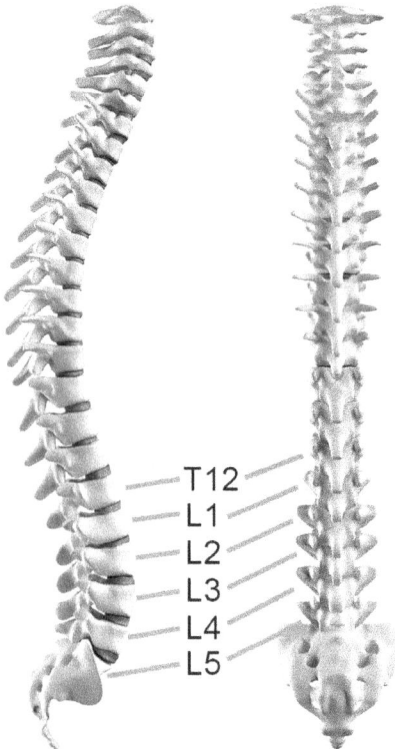

Where You Feel the Pain

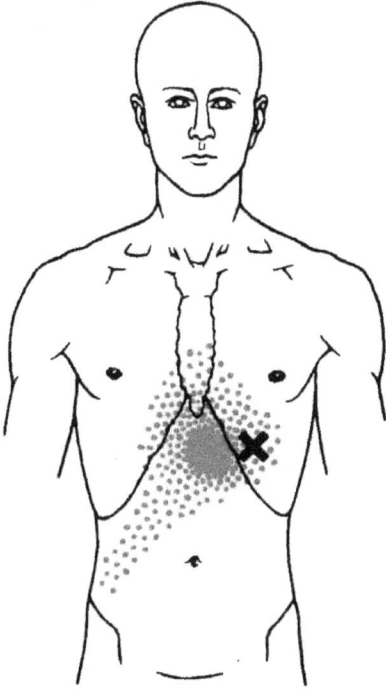

External oblique   **External oblique**

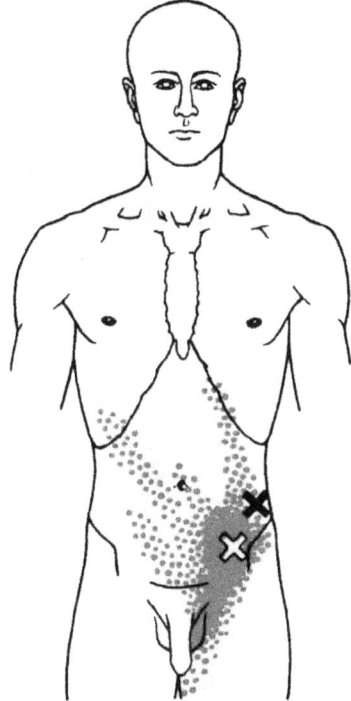

From Travell and Simmons' *Myofascial Pain and Dysfunction: The Trigger Point Manual V. 1 and 2* Copyright © 1998 and 1992 by Wolters Kluwer Brown.

A spasm in the abdominal oblique muscles usually refer pain to the front of the body, pelvis, and hip.

How to Perform the Release

Perform the release for both sides of the body if you feel tenderness in both tender points.

Most muscles only have one position to release the muscle spasm, but the abdominal obliques have two different positions you can try.

First, try **option 1**.

If the muscle spasm does not release, try **option 2**.

The tender point for the abdominal oblique muscles release is in the side of the body.

Find the Tender Point: Step 1

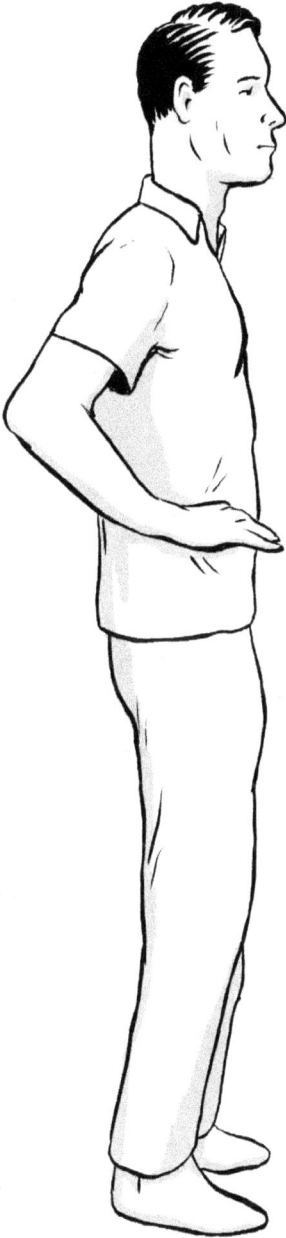

While in a standing position, place your thumb above your hip bone from the side.

Press your thumb into the middle of the body, in the space between the top of the hip and the bottom of the rib.

If the muscle is ticklish or painful, it is in spasm.

Find the Tender Point: Step 2

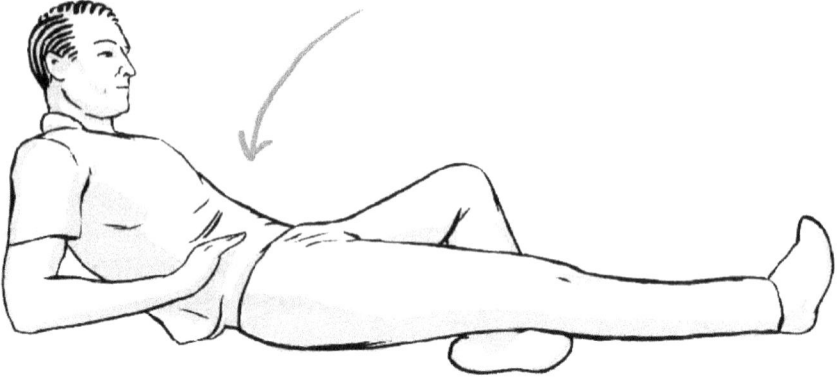

Keep the thumb in place.
  Change position to the back.

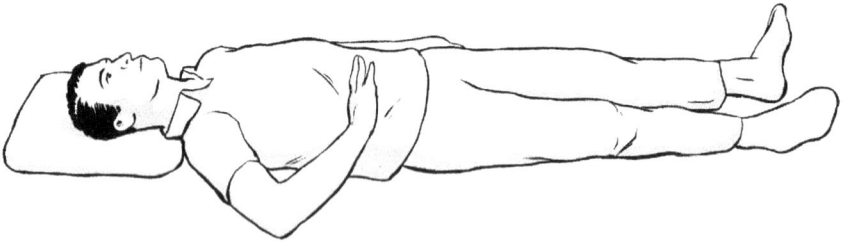

Lie on your back with your legs straight. Keep your thumb on the tender point with a light touch.
  You should be relaxed and comfortable.

Options

Now that you have located the tender point, it's time to get into position.

First, try the position of **option 1**.

If the muscle spasm does not release, try **option 2**.

Option 1

Get Into Position: Step 1

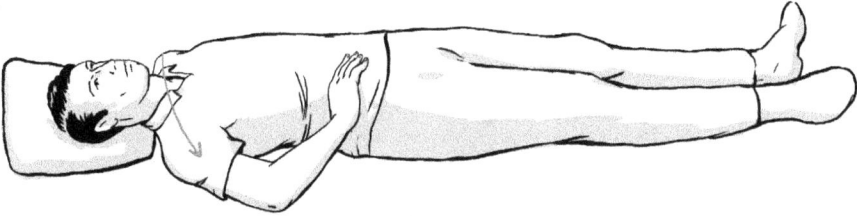

Slide your shoulders slightly in the direction of the tender point.

Don't shrug your shoulders. Instead, hinge from the waist.

Get Into Position: Step 2

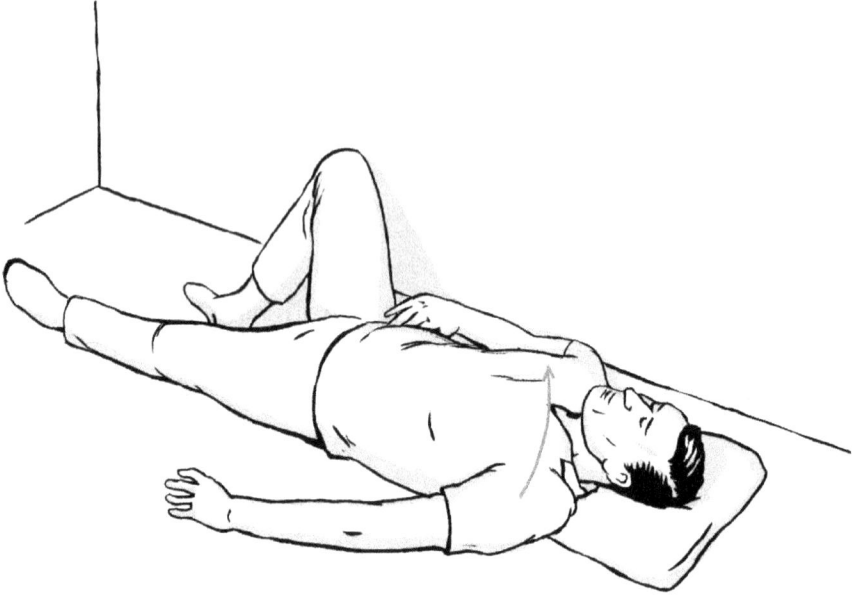

Bend your knee to the side at a 45-degree angle to the floor, and lay it on a pillow, or against a couch or a wall.

Get Into Position: Step 3

Your body must be in the correct position for the muscle release to take place, so you will now use the tender point to find out if you have placed your body in the correct position.

Make 2 deep pokes in the tender point.

If your body is in the correct position, the tender point will be 60–70% softer, or less tender and painful, or both, than the first time you poked in this spot.

If you are not in the correct position, adjust your body slightly. Move your knee up or down, or left or right, then after each adjustment check the tender point with 1 deep poke.

Continue to adjust your body position until the tender point is 60–70% softer, or less tender and painful, or both, than the first time you poked in this spot.

Get Into Position: Step 4

If you are not in the correct position, make slight adjustments to your knee position.

1. Slide your knee toward the wall or away from it.

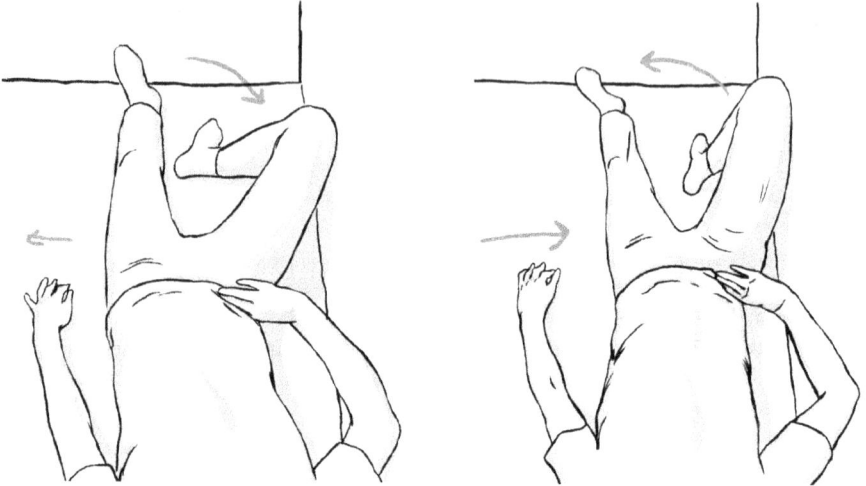

2. Slide your knee toward your face or away from it.

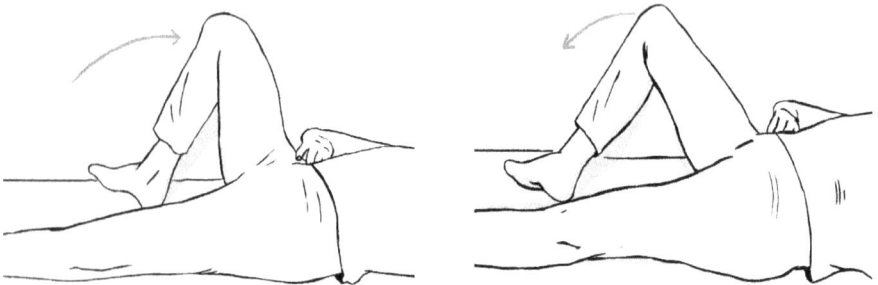

Perform the Release: Step 1

Once you have found the correct position, change finger pressure to a light touch.

Hold this touch and your body position for 90 seconds.

Perform the Release: Step 2

After holding for 90 seconds, make 2 deep pokes into the tender point.

It should be 60–70% less tender and painful, softer, or both.

Quality Check

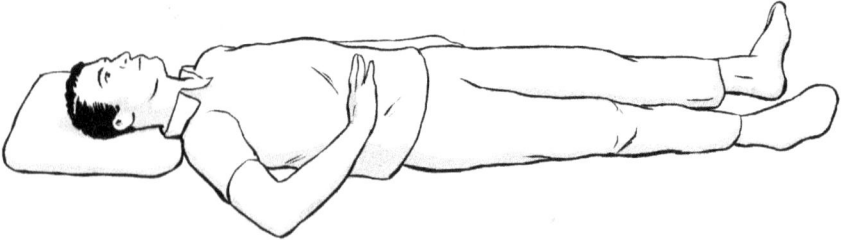

Keep a light touch on the point as you return to neutral position. Slide your knee back to center and straighten your leg.

Slide your shoulders back to center.

Check the tender point one last time to confirm that the release was successfully executed. It should still be at least 60–70% softer, or less tender and painful or both. This is the real test to determine if the spasm has been released.

Option 2

Get Into Position: Step 1

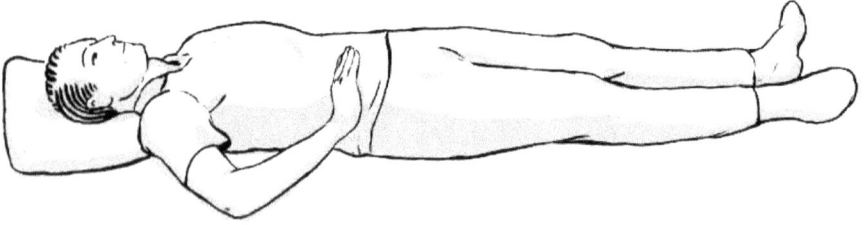

Keep finger pressure to a light touch, just to maintain location of the tender point.

Lie on the floor, on your back.

Get Into Position: Step 2

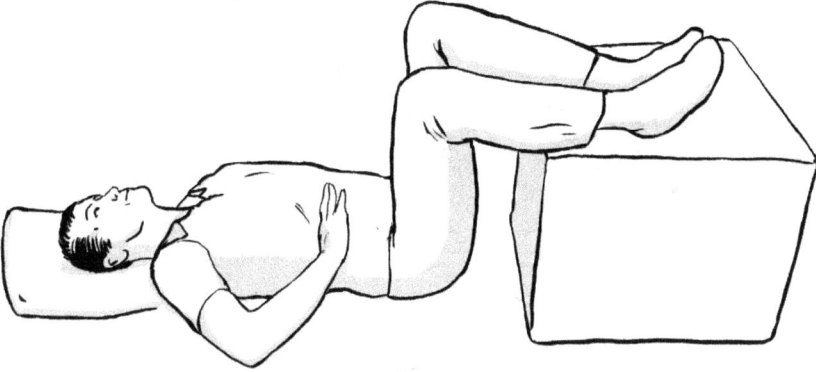

One foot at a time, place both feet on the seat of a couch or on a large foam block.

Knees are bent at 90–100 degrees to the floor.

Get Into Position: Step 3

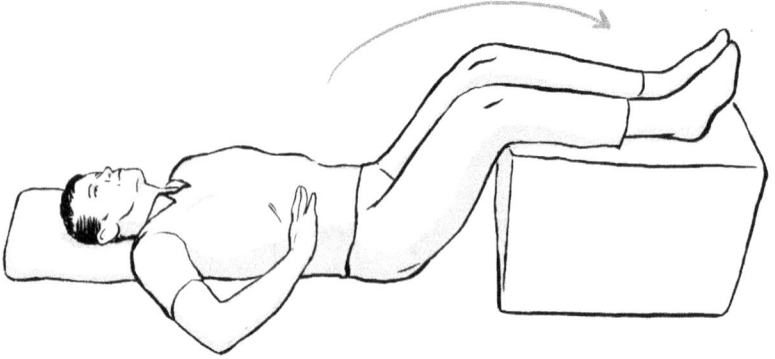

Push your feet and knees forward, away from your face.

In this position, you begin with legs bent at 90 degrees, and as you push forward, stop when the angle is 60–70 degrees.

Get Into Position: Step 4

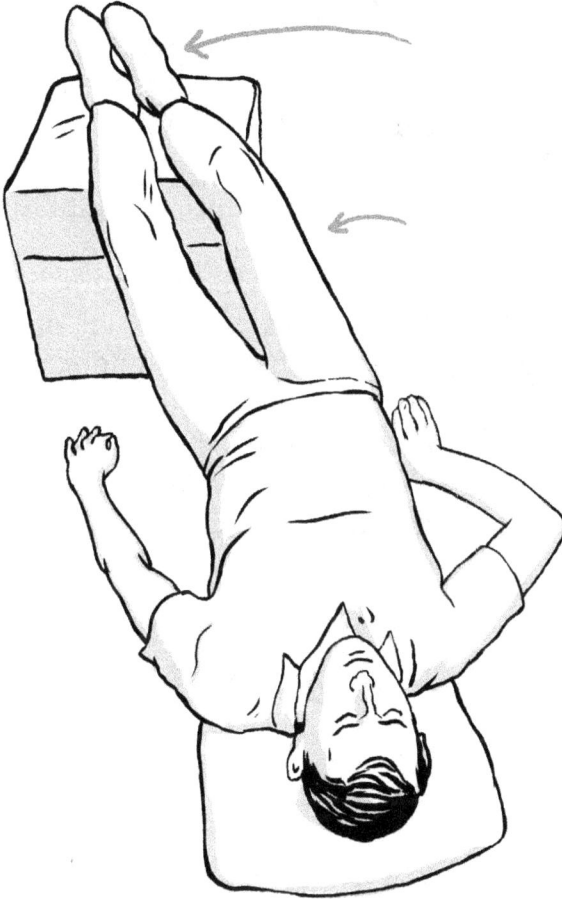

If you are working the right-side tender point, slide knees to the left.

If you're working the left-side tender point, slide knees to the right.

Knees are still around 60–70 degrees.

Get Into Position: Step 5

Your body must be in the correct position for the muscle release to take place, so you will now use the tender point to find out if you have placed your body in the correct position.

Make 2 deep pokes in the tender point.

If your body is in the correct position, the tender point will be 60–70% softer, or less tender and painful, or both, than the first time you poked in this spot.

If you are not in the correct position, adjust your body slightly. For example, move your knees up or down, or left or right, then after each adjustment check the tender point with 1 deep poke.

Continue to adjust your body position until the tender point is 60–70% softer, or less tender and painful, or both, than the first time you poked in this spot.

Perform the Release: Step 1

Once you have found the correct position, change finger pressure to a light touch. Hold this touch and your body position for 90 seconds.

Perform the Release: Step 2

After holding for 90 seconds, make 2 deep pokes into the tender point.

It should be 60–70% less tender and painful, softer, or both.

Quality Check

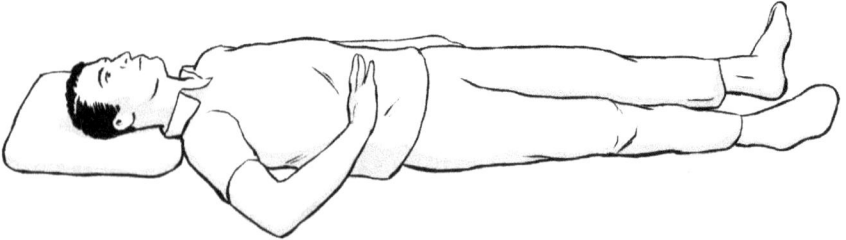

Keep a light touch on the point as you return to neutral position. Move one leg at a time, back to the floor and straighten them.

Check the tender point one last time with 2 deep pokes (not more than that) to confirm that the release was successfully executed. It should still be at least 60–70% softer, or less tender and painful or both.

This is the real test to determine if the spasm has been released.

Spinal

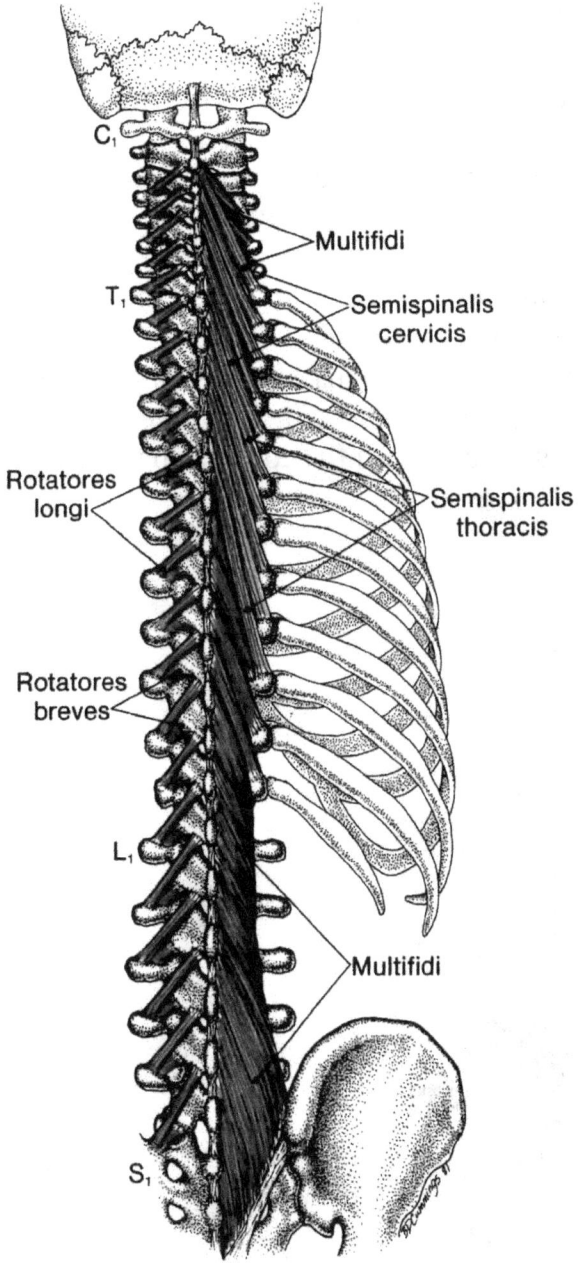

C₁

Multifidi

T₁

Semispinalis
cervicis

Rotatores
longi

Semispinalis
thoracis

Rotatores
breves

L₁

Multifidi

S₁

What You Need to Know

The spinal muscles are composed of three layers of muscles. Some muscles are close to the spine, while others are a bit farther away from it. Some are deep and some are superficial.

This group of overlapping muscles are responsible for holding the body upright all day.

These muscles are connected to the spine from top to bottom—as far down as the tailbone and as high up as the neck and the back of the head.

When the spinal muscles are in spasm, they can create restrictions in the vertebrae of the lower back (L1–L5).

This release focuses on the lower part of the muscles.

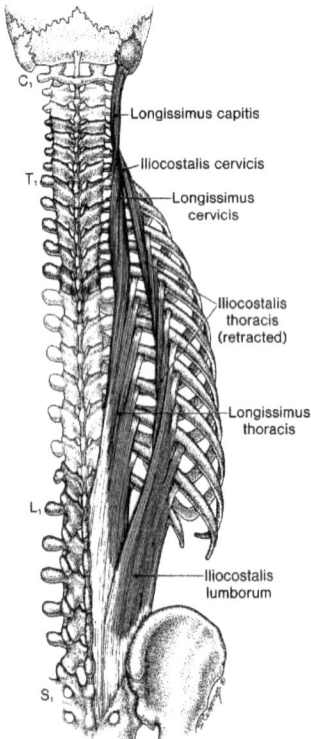

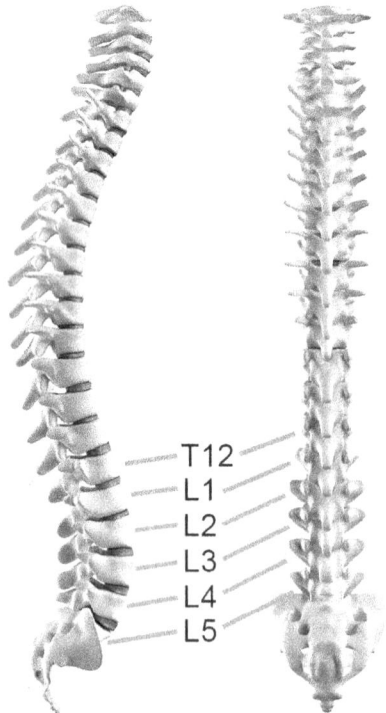

Where You Feel the Pain: 1

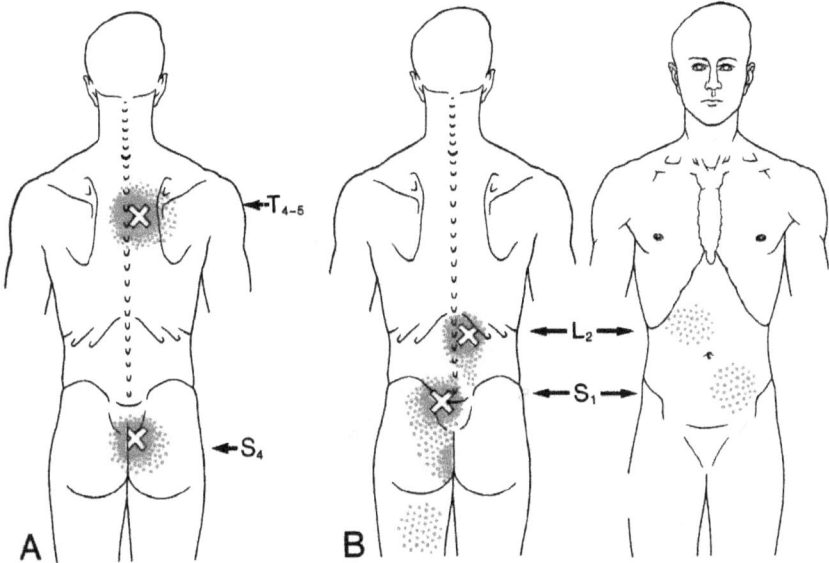

From Travell and Simmons' *Myofascial Pain and Dysfunction: The Trigger Point Manual V. 1 and 2* Copyright © 1998 and 1992 by Wolters Kluwer Brown.

When the spinal muscles are spastic, and the L1–L5 vertebrae are restricted, the pain is typically referred to the upper, lower back, and buttocks.

Where You Feel the Pain: 2

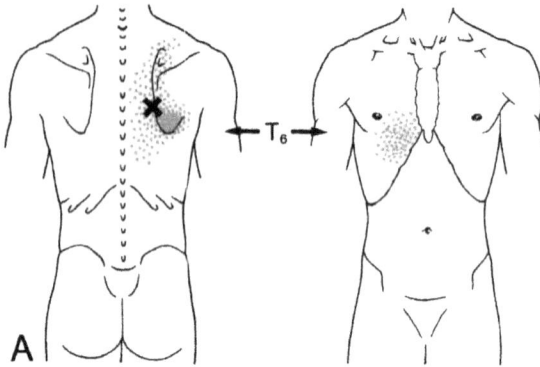

A Iliocostalis thoracis

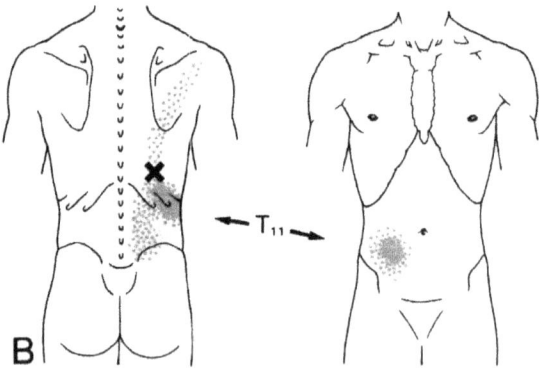

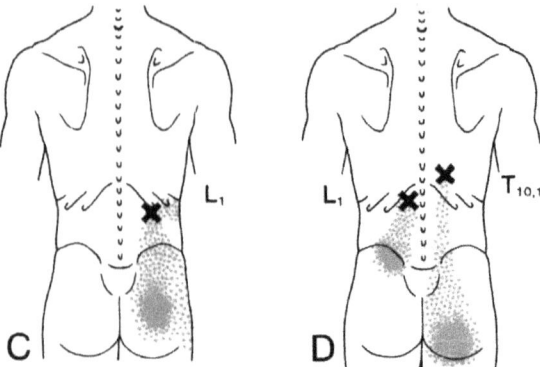

B Iliocostalis thoracis

C

D

From Travell and Simmons' *Myofascial Pain and Dysfunction: The Trigger Point Manual V. 1 and 2* Copyright © 1998 and 1992 by Wolters Kluwer Brown.

How to Perform the Release

Check the tender points on both sides of the body.

If the tender point is painful or tender, perform the release on that side.

Find the Tender Point: Step 1

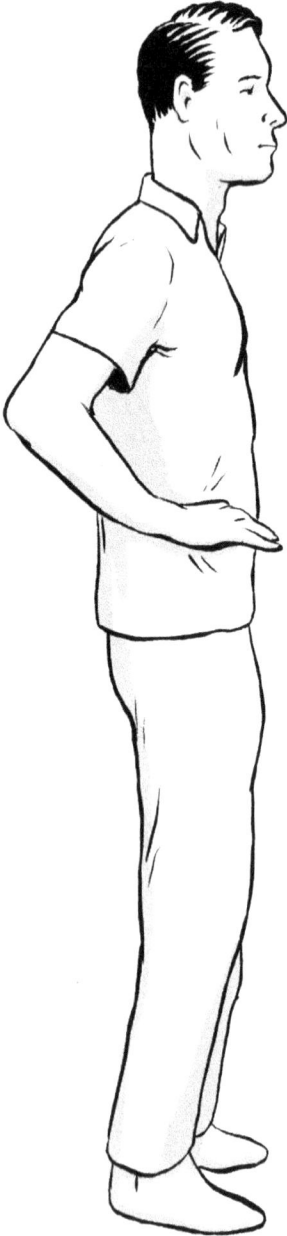

Stand relaxed.

Legs should be hip-width apart.

Place your hand on your hip so that your thumb is located on your back, between the rib cage and hip bone.

Find the Tender Point: Step 2

Slide your thumb toward the spine and stop when you touch it.

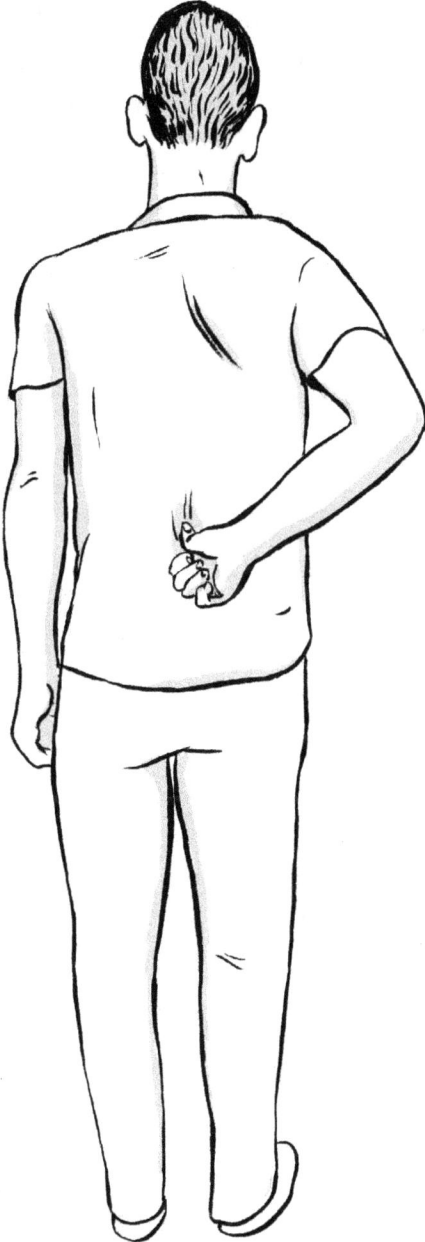

Find the Tender Point: Step 2.1

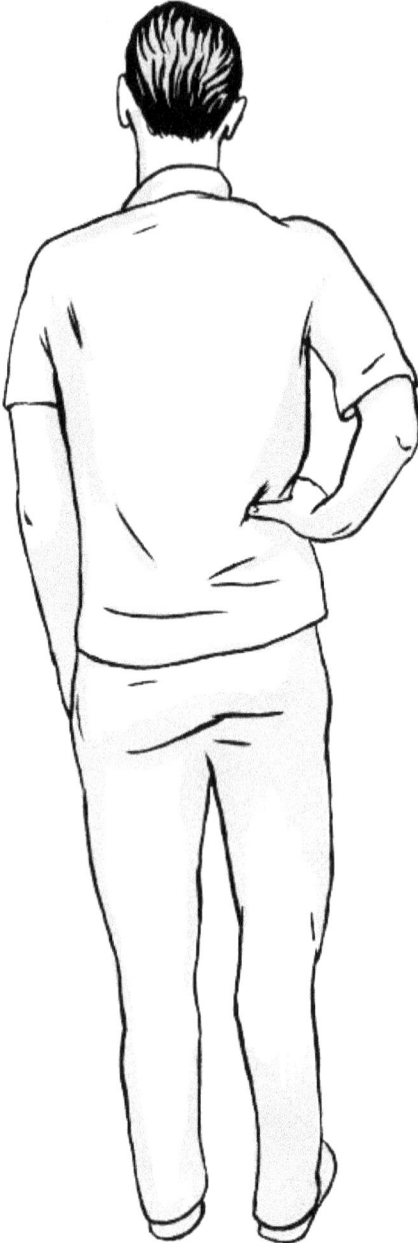

Next, slide your thumb 1–2 inches back (in the reverse direction) away from your spine.

You want your finger to be on the muscle, not the spine.

Find the Tender Point: Step 3

With your thumb still in position, 1–2 inches away from the spine, press your thumb straight into the muscle as if you are pushing forward toward the front of your body.

Press the thumb 1–2 times.

It may feel tender or painful.

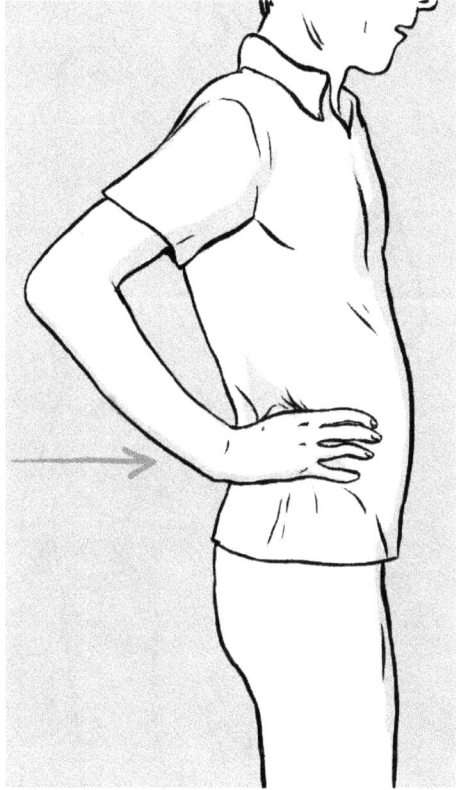

Get Into Position: Step 1

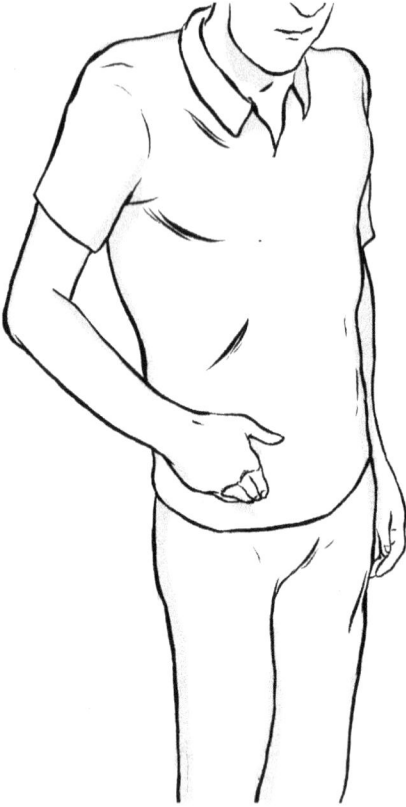

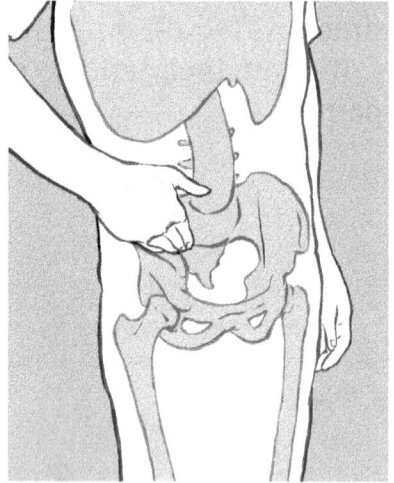

While standing, let go of the tender point and place your hand on the hip bone.

Place your fingers on the top-front part of the hip bone.

Get Into Position: Step 2

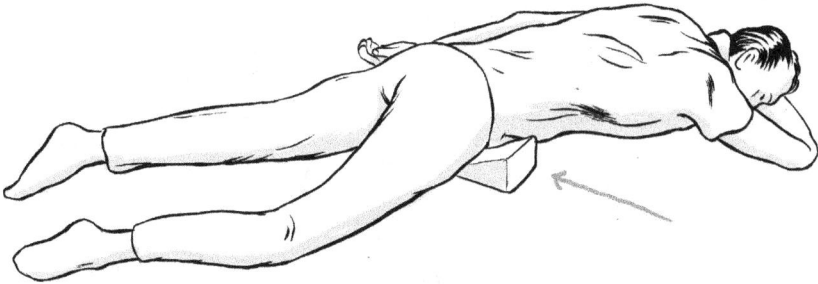

Lie on the floor, on your stomach.

Slide a small wedge (or an upside down boot) under the top-front part of the hip bone on the same side as the tender point you are working.

Get Into Position: Step 3.1

While lying face down, adjust the position of the wedge. It should be 45-degrees in the following two ways:

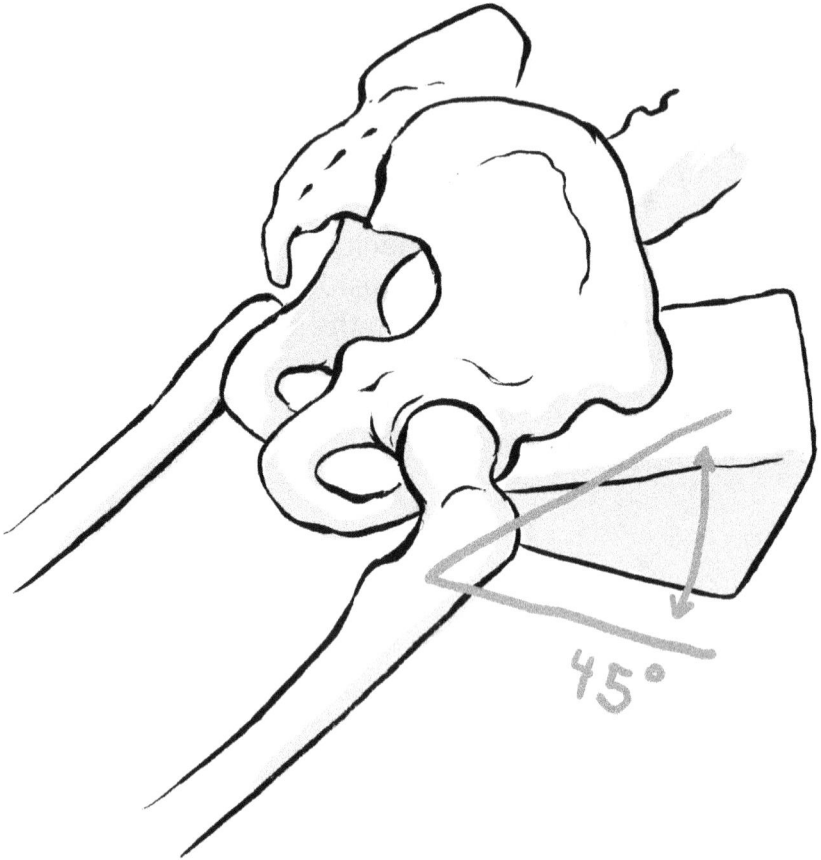

45°

The wedge raises your hip off the floor at 45-degrees.

Get Into Position: Step 3.2

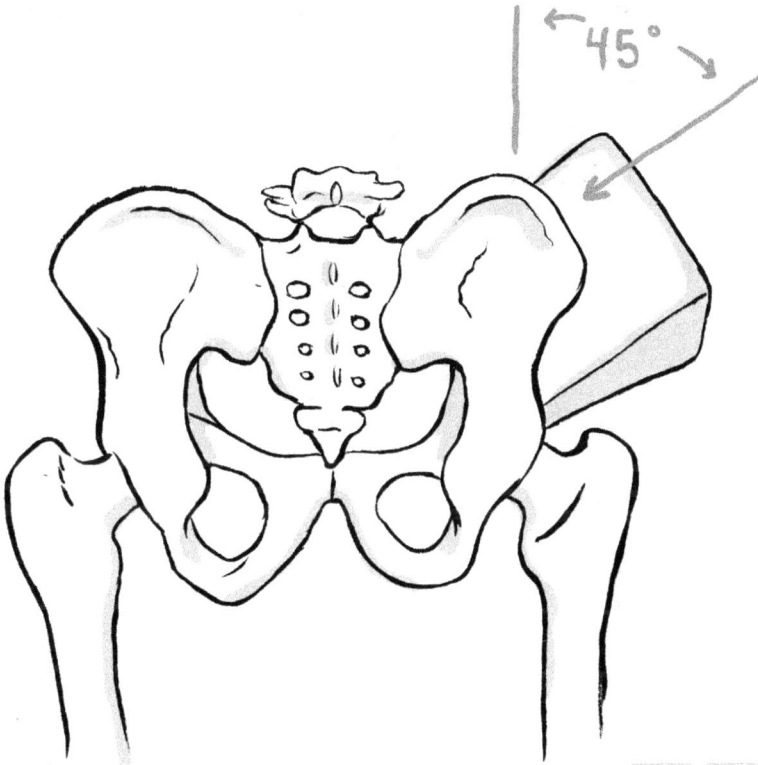

The wedge is placed under the hip bone at 45-degrees.

Get Into Position: Step 4

Once you are in position, it will be difficult to check the tender point again.

Instead of checking the tender point, make sure your position feels comfortable. If not, make slight adjustments to the wedge. For example, push it inward to elevate the hip, or pull it out to lower the hip.

Remember: your body must be in the correct position for the release to take place.

Perform the Release: Step 1

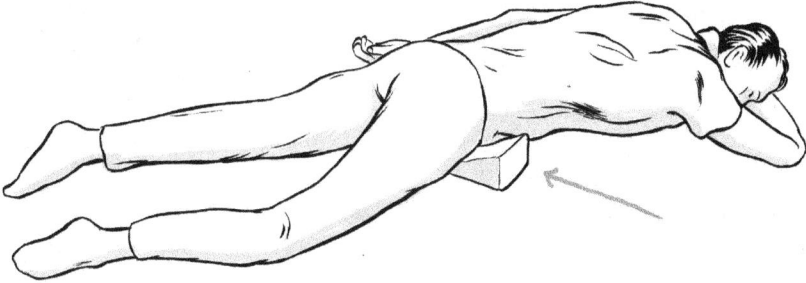

Hold your body in position for 90 seconds. This is when the muscle release occurs.

The position should be passive and comfortable with no effort.

You must be relaxed and must not use your muscles to hold yourself in place.

Do not move your body.

Quality Check

Return to neutral in a standing position.

Check the tender point one last time with 2 deep pokes to confirm that the release was successfully executed.

This is the real test to determine if the spasm has been released.

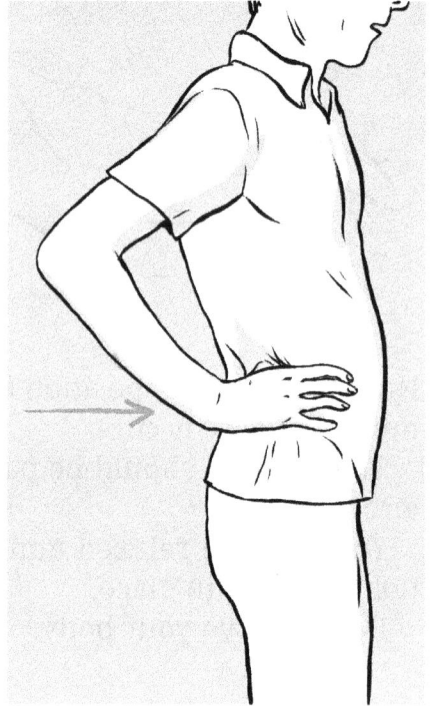

Secondary Release

There is a secondary and optional release available for the spinal muscles in the lower back.

With this release, there is no tender point to check, so you will not have to keep your finger on a point.

You will need to use a sofa or a chair. Choose one with a seat that is the height of your lower back, while you are kneeling on your knees.

WARNING

Do not use this release if you have complications with a disc, such as a herniatiated disc or impinged nerve.

Perform the Release: Step 1

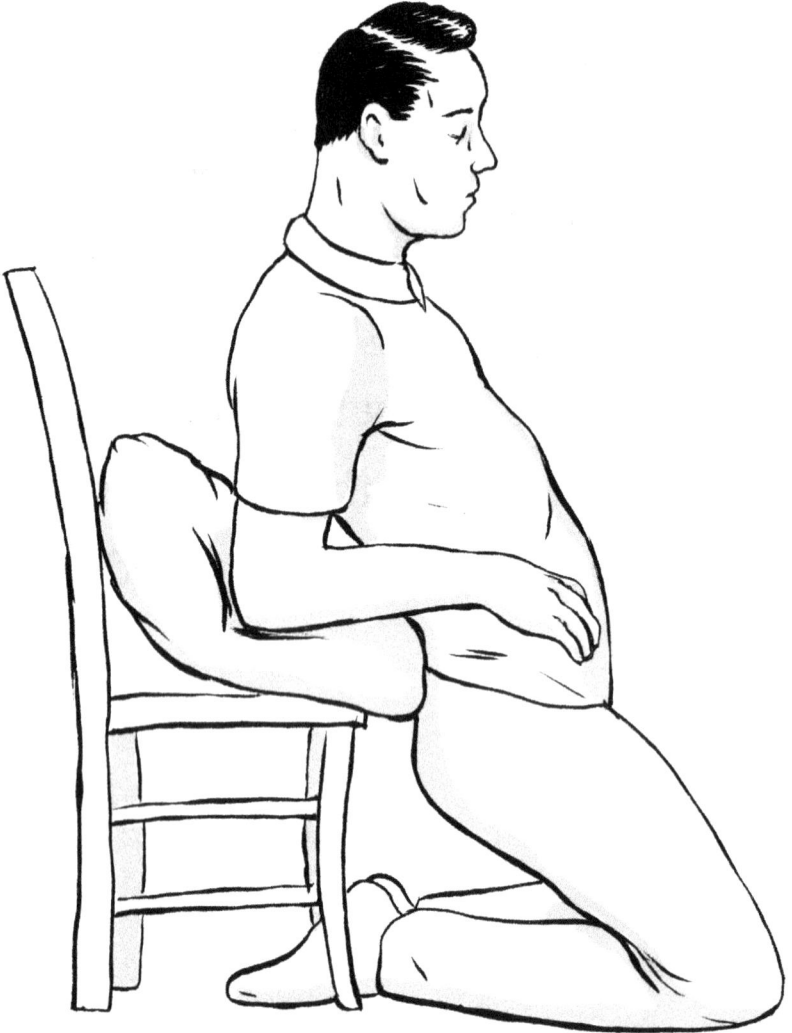

Sit on your knees.
　　Place your lower back on the edge of the sofa or chair.
　　Support yourself on your bent elbows.

Perform the Release: Step 2

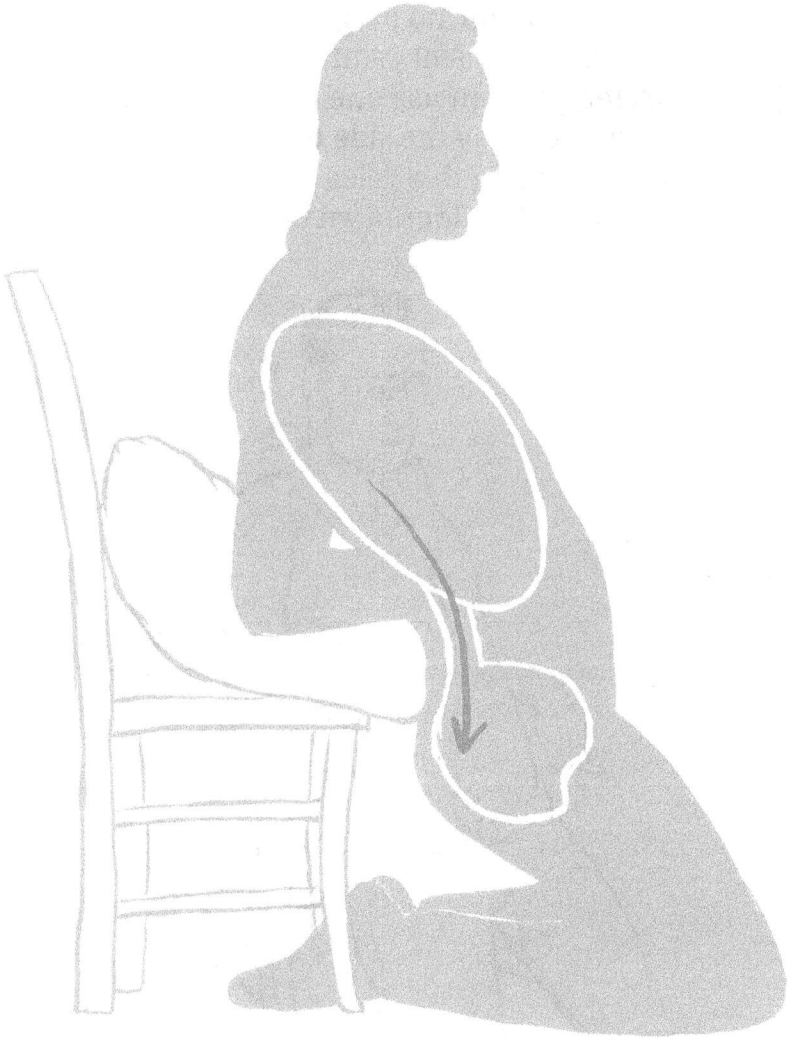

Next, you're going to relax your lower back muscles.
Start by pushing your abdomen forward. This will create a sway in the lower back by tipping the pelvis forward and shifting your weight to the elbows.

You will feel your lower back muscles slacken. Do not use them to hold up your body weight.

Perform the Release: Step 3

Stay in this position for no longer than 20 seconds.

The position should feel comfortable. If not, stop.

If you prefer, you can use one knee on the floor at a time, instead of both. Choose the side that is most comfortable to you when performing this release. The other leg's foot will then be placed on the floor at an almost 90 degree angle.

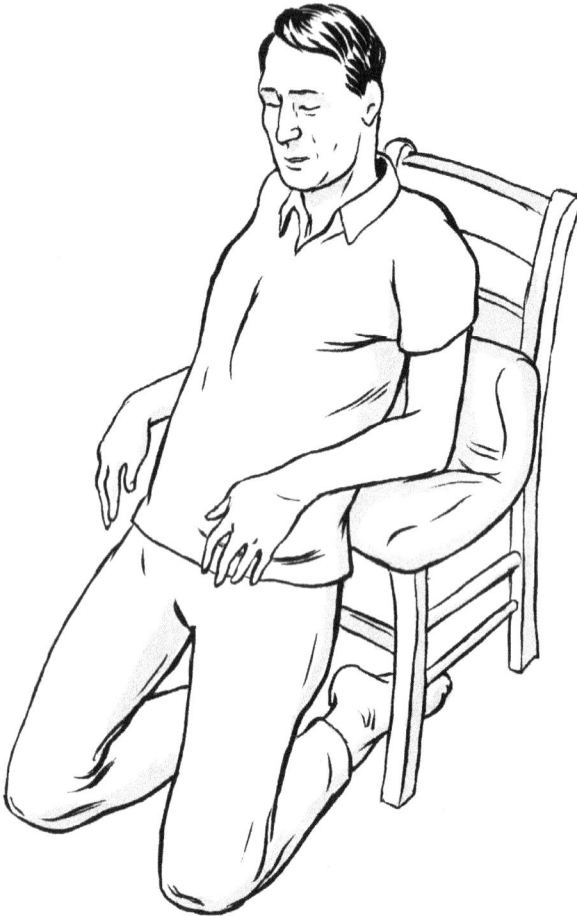

Get up slowly and carefully.

Quality Check

Return to neutral in a standing position.

Check the tender point one last time with 2 deep pokes into the side muscle of the spine in the lower back.

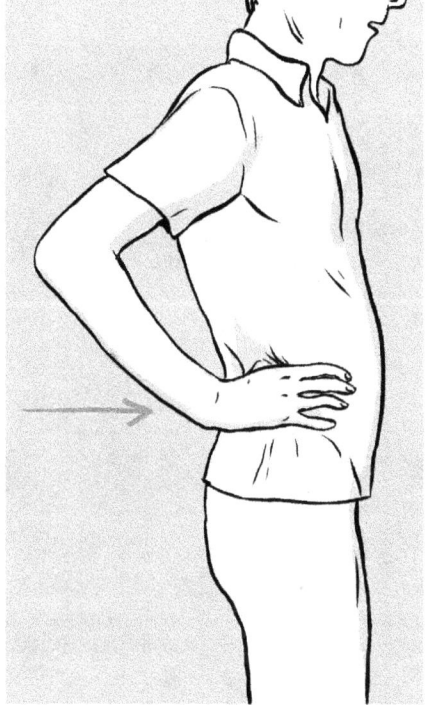

Quadratus Lumborum

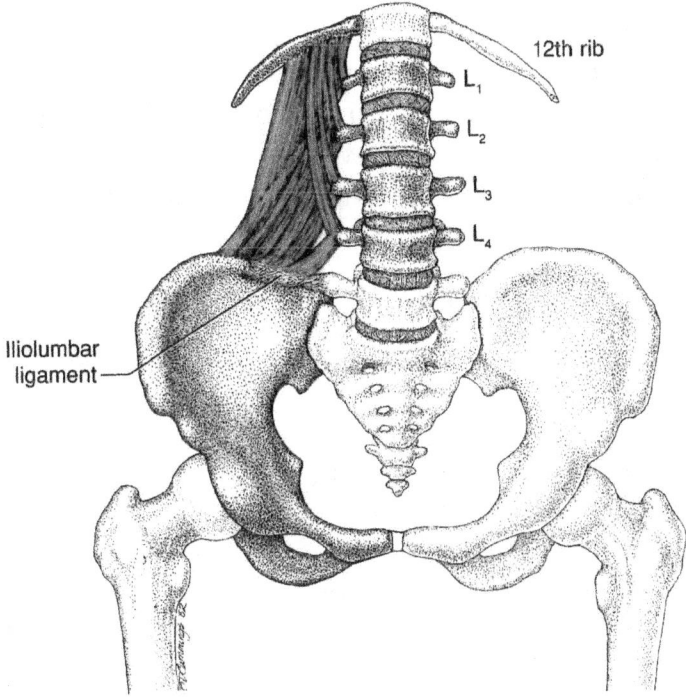

12th rib

L₁

L₂

L₃

L₄

Iliolumbar
ligament

What You Need to Know

The quadratus lumborum (QL) muscle is attached to the sides of the spine, to the last rib of the rib cage and to the superior part of the hip—all on the back side of the body.

For anyone whose hips are not level, which is common, you tend to compensate more with this muscle. One of its primary functions is to lift the hip. It's often referred to as the hip hiker.

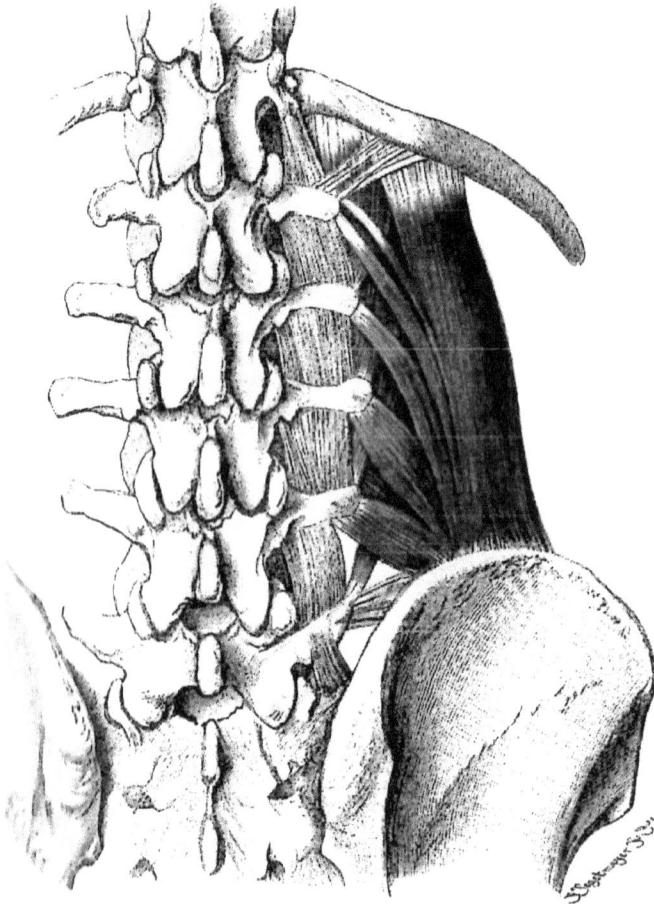

Where You Feel the Pain

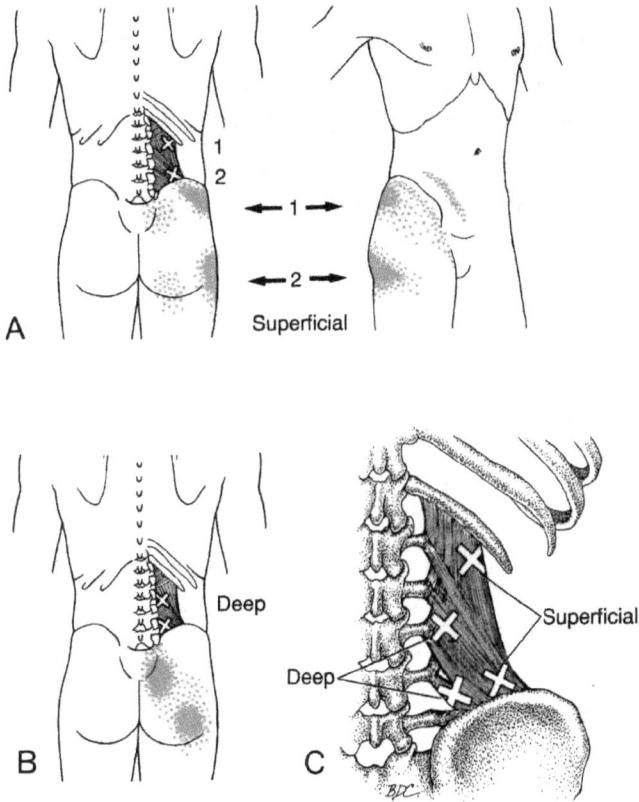

From Travell and Simmons' *Myofascial Pain and Dysfunction: The Trigger Point Manual V. 1 and 2* Copyright © 1998 and 1992 by Wolters Kluwer Brown.

A spastic quadratus lumborum muscle causes pain across the lower back, the lower buttocks, the hip, down the back of the thigh, and sometimes into the calf.

Often this pain is misdiagnosed as a sciatica problem, but it could very well be caused by a spastic QL.

How to Perform the Release

Perform the release for both sides of the body.

The QL muscle has several tender points because it is connected to the rib, the spine and the upper part of the hip. Two of them are described here, so be sure to try both tender points. For many people, the QL muscle is the main source of lower back pain, so it's important that this muscle is not missed.

Find the Tender Point: Step 1

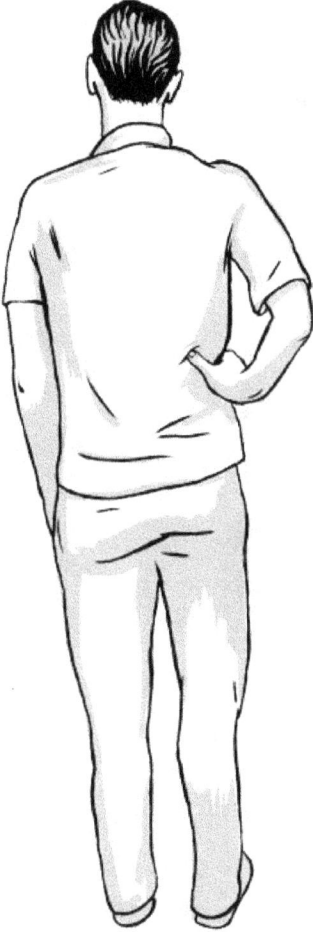

Stand relaxed, with your arms at your side. Next, place your thumb on the underside of the last rib.

Slide your thumb along the rib bone (which is at a 45-degree angle) toward the center of your body until you hit a muscle mass. This is the QL.

Once you hit the muscle mass, deep poke twice. Press deep into the muscle to locate the tender point. It will feel tender, painful, or resistant to the touch. When you poke, the pressure should be 4 times harder than a light poke.

A tender point is about 1 inch (2½ cm) in diameter under your finger.

Find the Tender Point: Step 2

To check the second tender point location, turn your thumb to 90 degrees (parallel to the floor).

Deep poke twice.

Press deep into the muscle to locate the tender point. It will feel tender, painful, or resistant to the touch. When you poke, the pressure should be 4 times harder than a light poke.

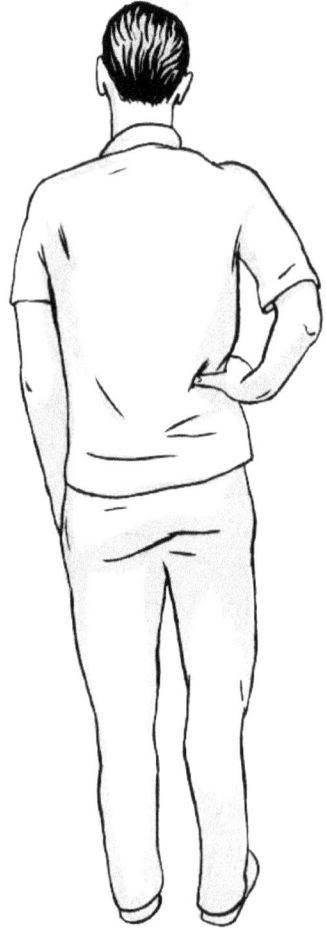

Find the Tender Point: Step 3

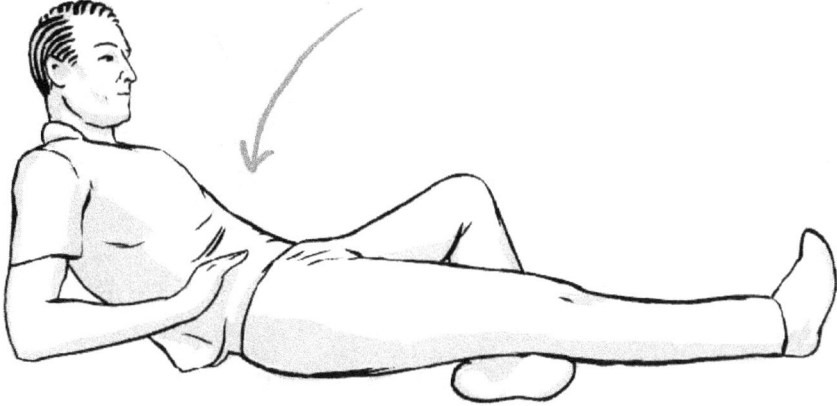

Once you have found the correct position, change finger pressure to a light touch, just to maintain location of the tender point.

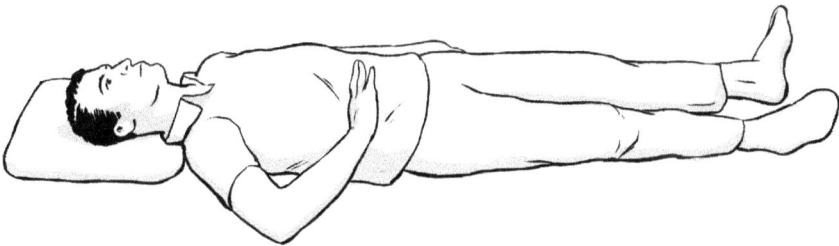

Keep the finger on the tender point while you change from a standing to a lying position on your back.

Get Into Position: Step 1

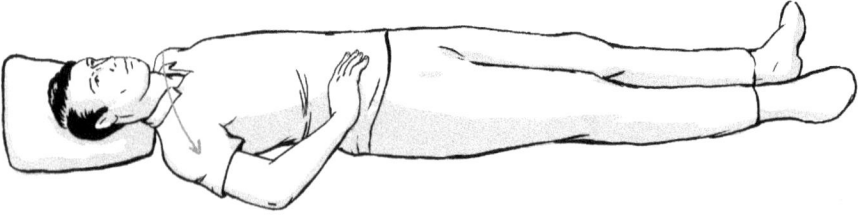

Slide your shoulders slightly in the direction of the tender point.

You can use another finger if it is more comfortable.

Get Into Position: Step 2

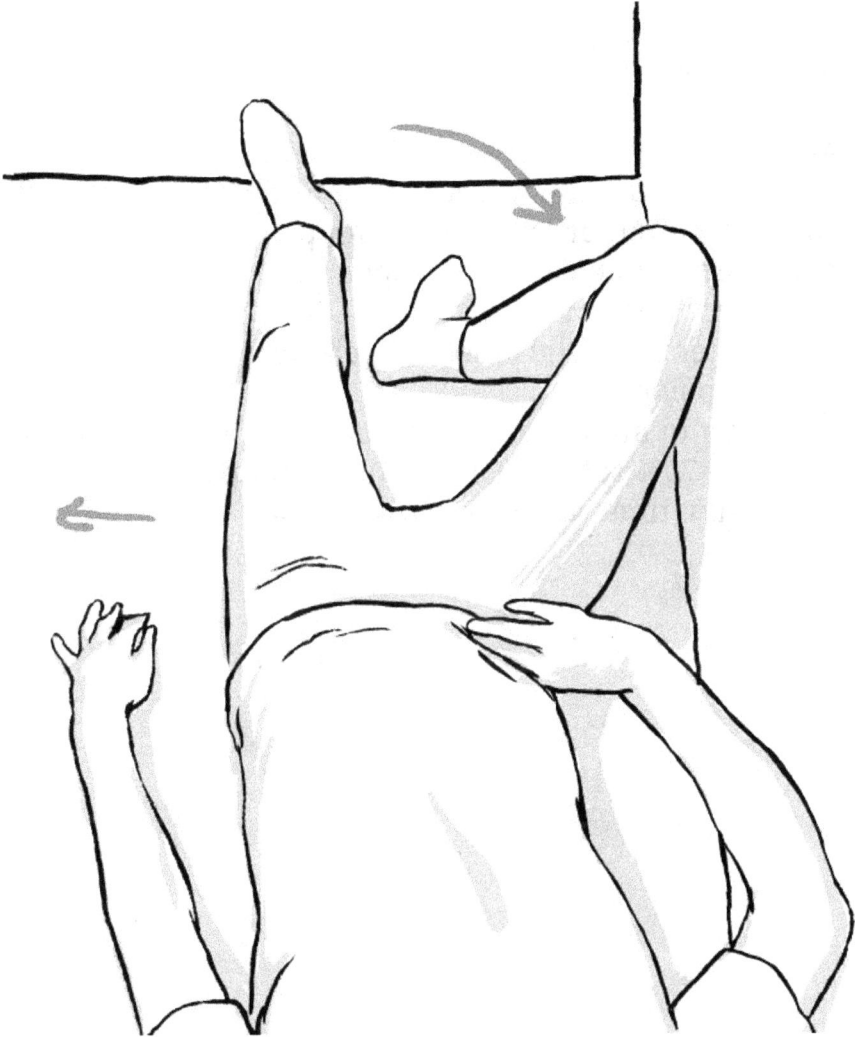

Bend your knee to the side at a 45-degree angle to the floor, and lay it on a pillow, or against a couch or a wall.

Get Into Position: Step 3

Your body must be in the correct position for the muscle release to take place, so you will now use the tender point to find out if you have placed your body in the correct position.

Make 2 deep pokes in the tender point.

If your body is in the correct position, the tender point will be 60–70% softer, or less tender and painful, or both, than the first time you poked in this spot.

If you are not in the correct position, adjust your body slightly. After each adjustment, check the tender point again with 1 deep poke.

Continue to adjust your body position until the tender point is 60–70% softer, or less tender and painful, or both, than the first time you poked in this spot.

Get Into Position: Step 4

If you are not in the correct position, make slight adjustments to your knee position.

1. Slide your knee toward the wall or away from it.

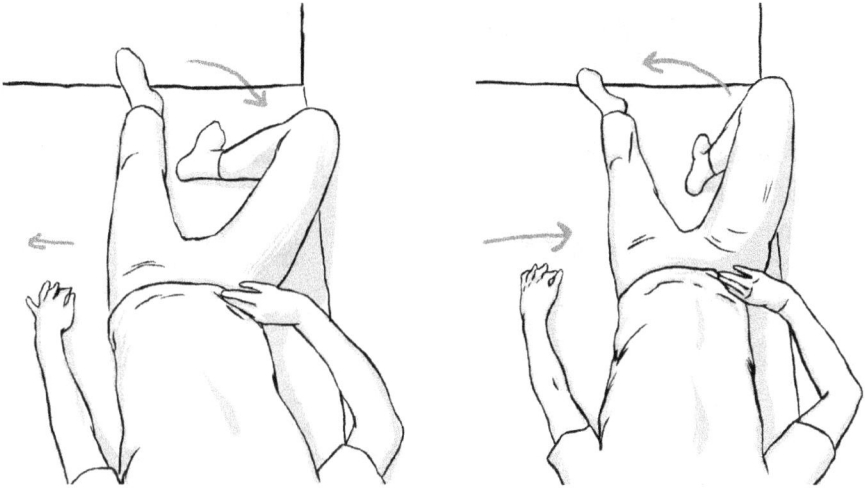

2. Slide your knee toward your face or away from it.

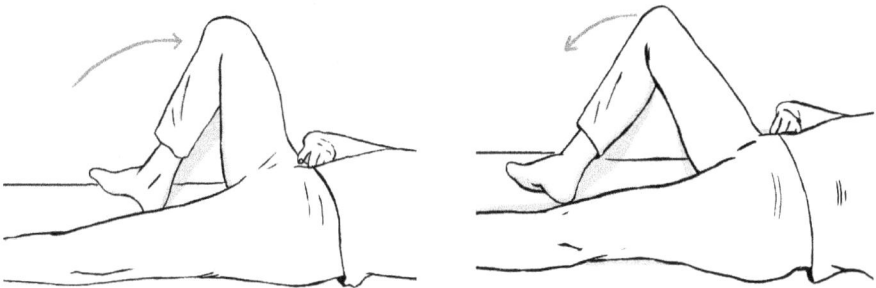

Perform the Release: Step 1

Once you have found the correct position, change finger pressure to a light touch.

Hold this touch and your body position for 90 seconds.

Perform the Release: Step 2

After holding for 90 seconds, make 2 deep pokes into the tender point.

It should be 60–70% less tender, painful, softer or both.

Quality Check

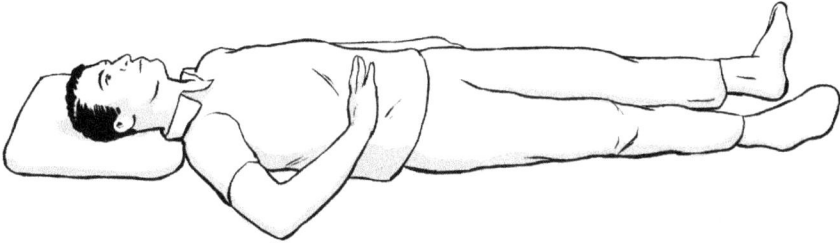

Keep a light touch on the point as you return to neutral position. Slide your knee back to center and straighten your leg.

Slide your shoulders back to center.

Check the tender point one last time to confirm that the release was successfully executed. It should still be at least 60–70% softer, or less tender and painful or both. This is the real test to determine if the spasm has been released.

Piriformis

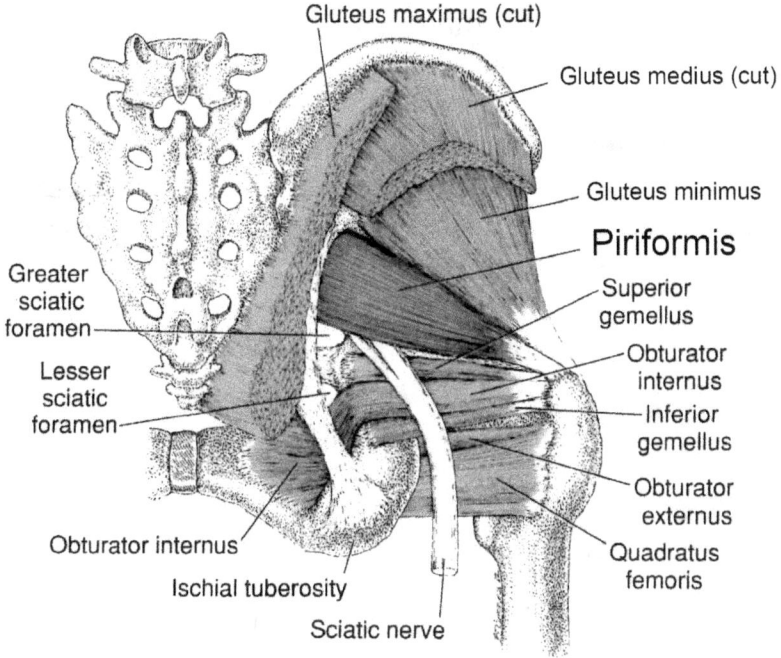

Gluteus maximus (cut)

Gluteus medius (cut)

Gluteus minimus

Piriformis

Greater sciatic foramen

Superior gemellus

Obturator internus

Lesser sciatic foramen

Inferior gemellus

Obturator externus

Obturator internus

Quadratus femoris

Ischial tuberosity

Sciatic nerve

What You Need to Know

The piriformis muscle is located in the buttocks. It is located between the tail bone and the hip joint and crosses over the buttocks at a 45-degree angle.

It is one of the deep muscles of the gluteal. It's the third layer: first there's the gluteus maximus, then the gluteus medius and minimus, and the third layer includes the piriformis, which is responsible for external rotation of the hip, along with a few other muscles.

Where You Feel the Pain

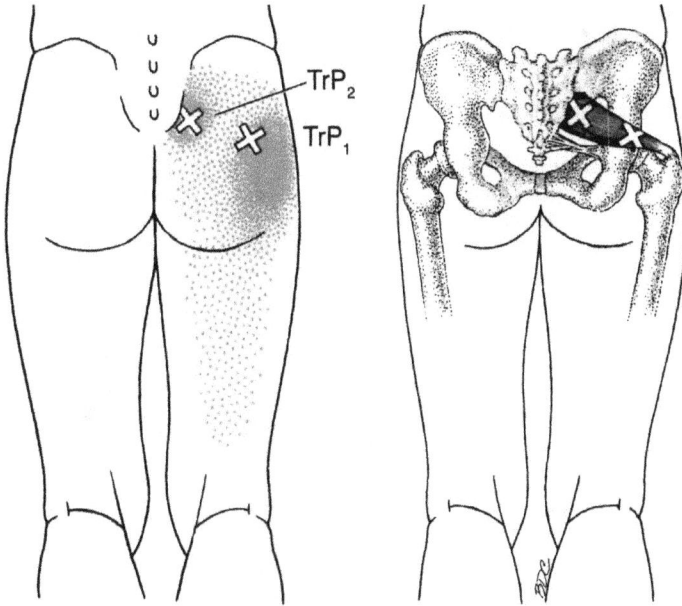

From Travell and Simmons' *Myofascial Pain and Dysfunction: The Trigger Point Manual V. 1 and 2* Copyright © 1998 and 1992 by Wolters Kluwer Brown.

A spastic piriformis muscle causes a shooting pain to the lower back, buttocks and hip, and can mimic the symptoms of the sciatic nerve by entrapping the nerve and creating numbness and tingling down the back of the thigh, calf and sole of the foot. The pain can be severe and debilitating.

How to Perform the Release

First check the tender point on the side of the body where you feel the most referred pain.

If the tender point is painful, do the release on that side. If the tender point is not painful, then don't do the release.

Find the Tender Point: Step 1

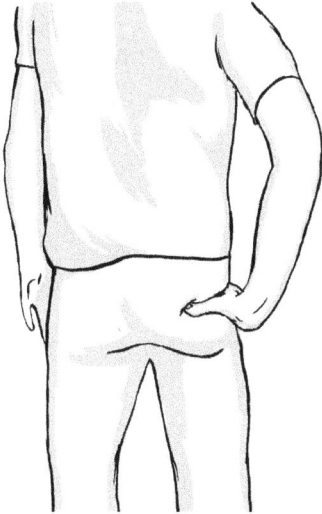

Stand relaxed, with your arms at your side.

Put your finger on the side of your tail bone. Slide your finger outward and downward at a 45-degree angle toward the hip joint. Stop when you find the halfway point between the tail bone and the hip joint.

The tender point is in the center of the gluteus muscle.

Deep poke 2 times. When you poke, the pressure should be 4 times harder than a light poke. It should feel tender, painful, or resistant to the touch. Sometimes, it will feel like a cable.

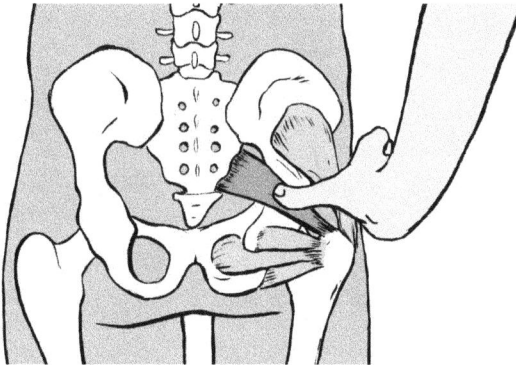

A tender point is about 1 inch (2½ cm) in diameter under your finger.

Find the Tender Point: Step 2

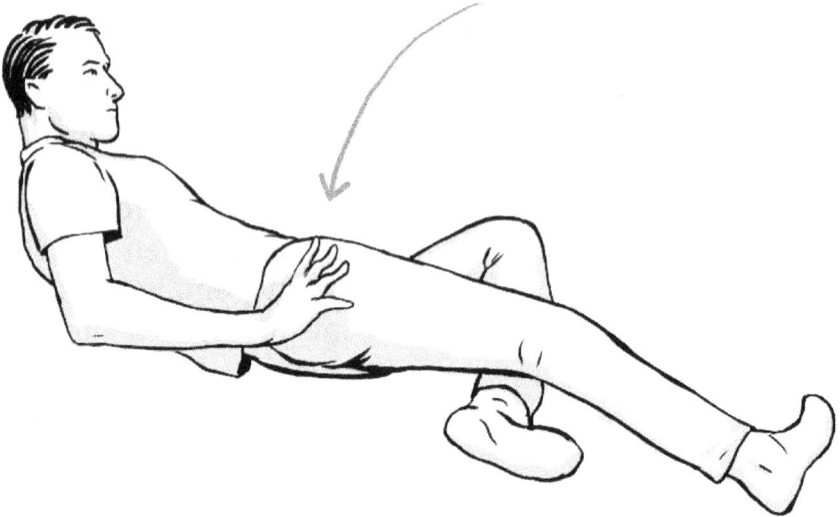

Change finger pressure to a light touch, just to maintain location of the tender point.

Keep the finger on the tender point while you change from a standing to a lying position on your back.

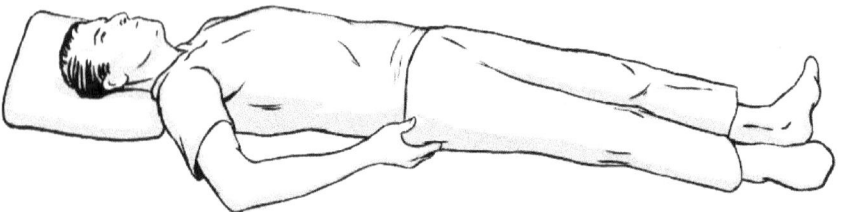

If it's more comfortable, you use your index finger, instead of your thumb.

Get Into Position: Step 1

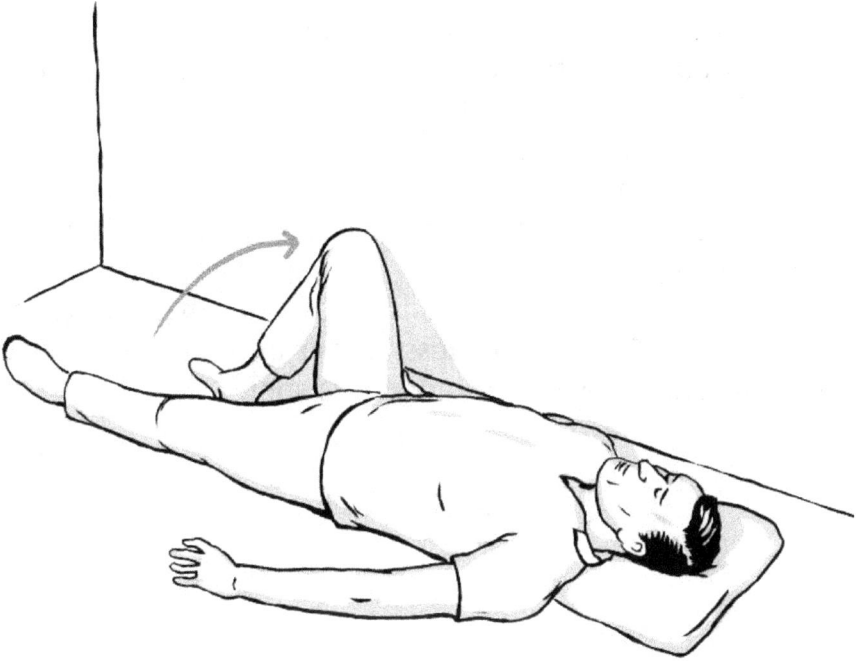

Lying on the floor, bend your knee, leaving the other leg straight.

Drop the knee outward to create a 45-degree angle with the floor.

Support the knee with a pillow, couch, foam block or wall.

Get Into Position: Step 2

Make 2 deep pokes in the tender point.

If your body is in the correct position, the tender point will be 60–70% softer, or less tender and painful, or both, than the first time you poked in this spot.

If you are not in the correct position, adjust your body slightly. After each adjustment, check the tender point again with 1 deep poke.

Continue to adjust your body position until the tender point is 60–70% softer, or less tender and painful, or both, than the first time you poked in this spot.

Get Into Position: Step 3

If you are not in the correct position, make slight adjustments to your knee position.

Slide your knee toward the wall or away from it.

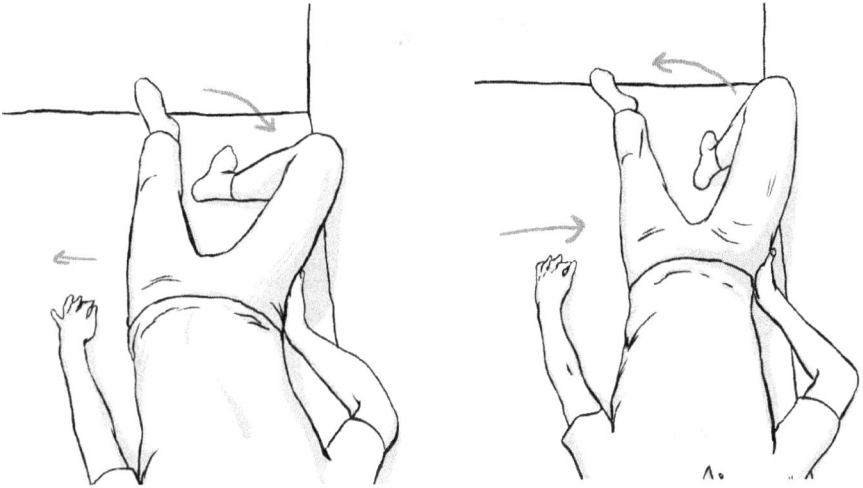

Slide your knee toward your face or away from it.

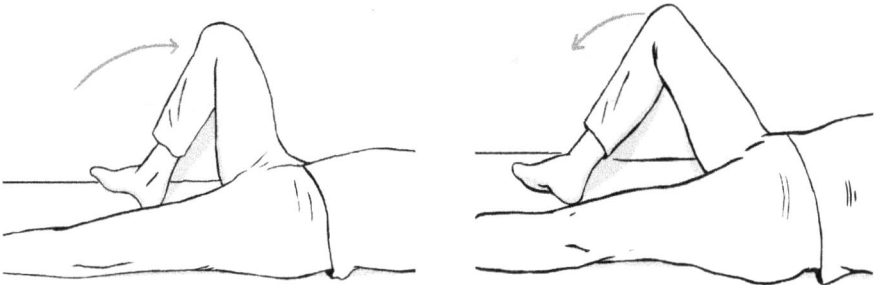

Perform the Release: Step 1

Once you have found the correct position, change finger pressure to a light touch.

Hold this touch and your body position for 90 seconds.

Perform the Release: Step 2

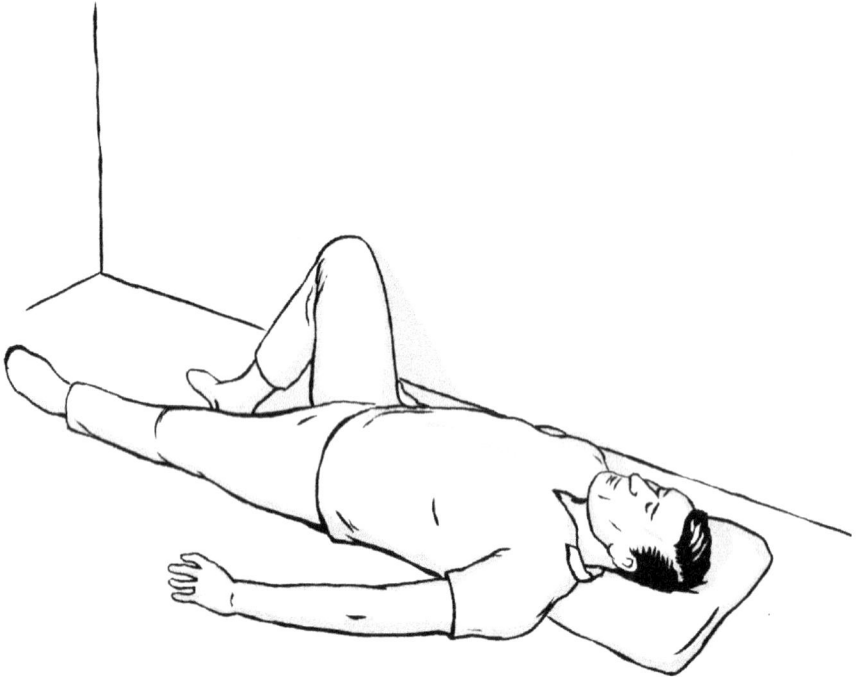

After holding for 90 seconds, make 2 deep pokes into the tender point.

It should be 60–70% less tender and painful, softer, or both.

Quality Check

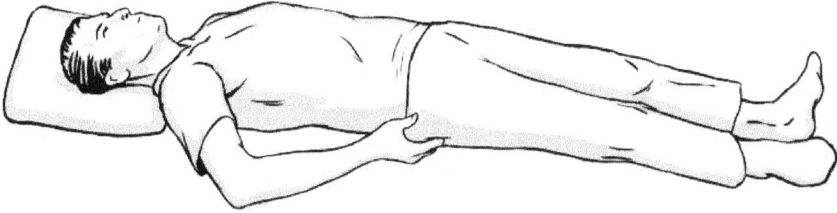

Keep a light touch on the point as you return to neutral position. Move one leg at a time, back to the floor, or bed, and straighten them.

Check the tender point one last time to confirm that the release was successfully executed. It should still be at least 60–70% softer, or less tender and painful or both. This is the real test to determine if the spasm has been released.

Conclusion

Congratulations, you have completed all the releases!

To maintain the benefits of these releases, be sure to scan and look for these tender points regularly—even if your lower back feels good, and you are not consciously aware of pain. Don't stop doing the release when you feel better. Keep doing it to prevent the muscles from becoming spastic again because we have to use the muscles all day long against gravity, and to maintain the health in your muscles.

The healing effect of this technique is cumulative. The more you do it, the more you supply the muscle with efficient circulation, and the easier it will be for the muscle to answer to the task it is being asked to do during the day. It will expand your safety zone, which is the time period in which you can do things without back pain.

If possible, do these releases at least 2 times a day. The more the better. The more you do them, the more efficient you will become. Over time, you will learn to trust your finger to find the tender points, and to find the correct position for the release. It all becomes easier in time.

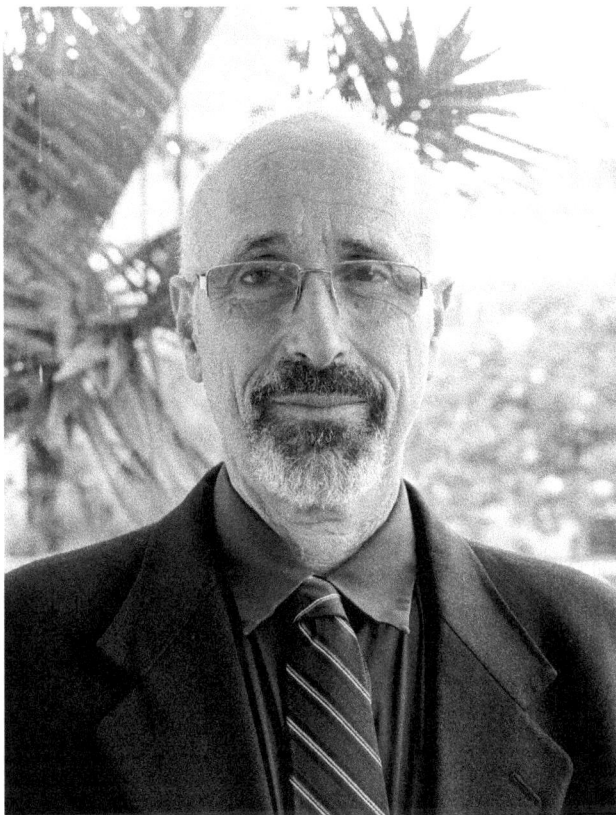

About the Author

Gadi Kaufman, NMT, JSCC, is a Certified Neuromuscular Therapist with a thriving private practice in Santa Monica, California. For more than 20 years, Gadi has provided relief of back pain for countless patients in Southern California. Gadi's approach to treatment focuses on the Strain Counterstrain technique, a unique and pain-free method for resetting the nervous system and releasing painful muscle spasms throughout the body. He has a degree in physical education, and certifications in neuromuscular therapy, applied kinesiology and Strain Counterstrain Technique.

Find more information about Gadi Kaufman and the Strain Counterstrain Technique at: *gadibody.com*.

Reference Guide

This is a quick reference guide that allows you to see the muscle, the tender point, and the positional release needed to bring you relief.

Psoas

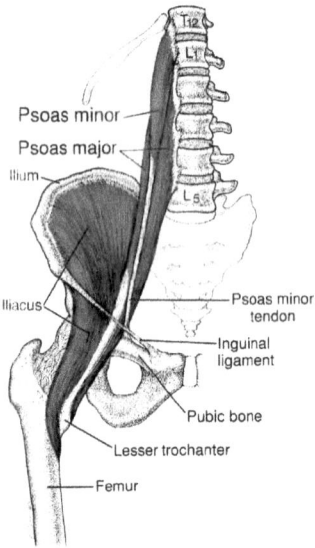

Page 1. Psoas

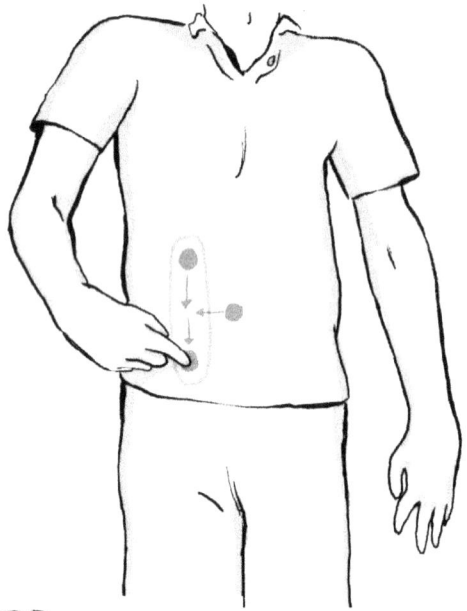

Page 8. Tender Points

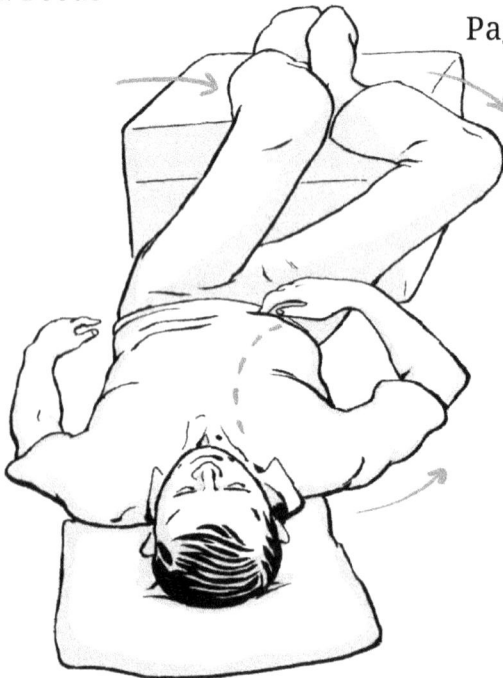

Page 12. Positional Release

Iliacus (Center)

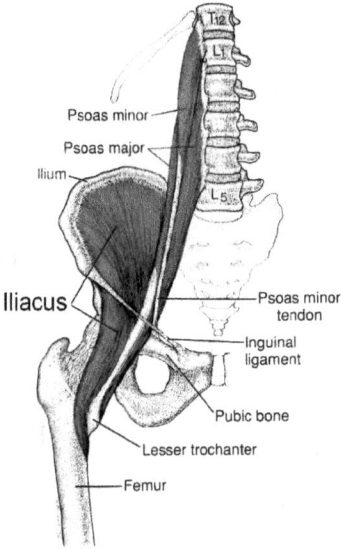

Page 17. Iliacus (Center)

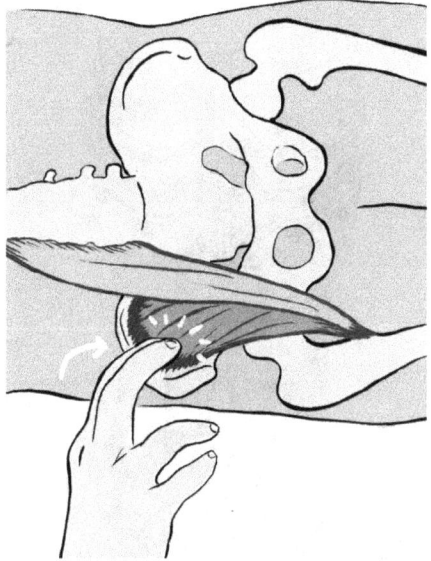

Page 23. Tender Points

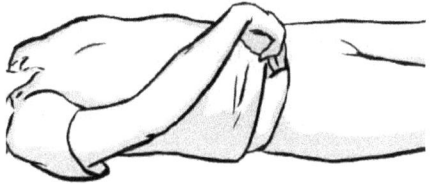

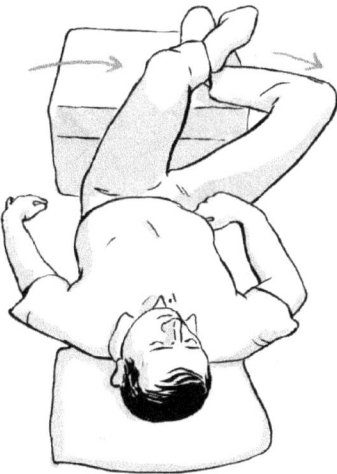

Page 27. Positional Release

Rectus Abdominus

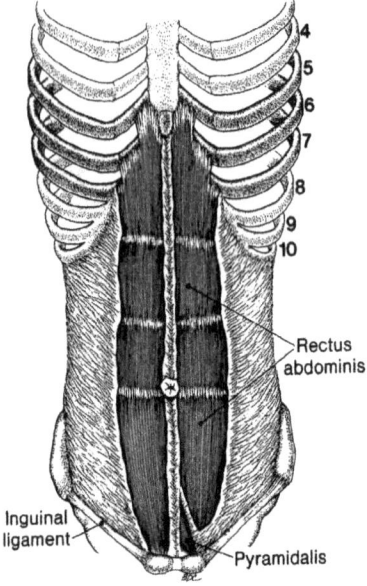

Page 31. Rectus Abdominus

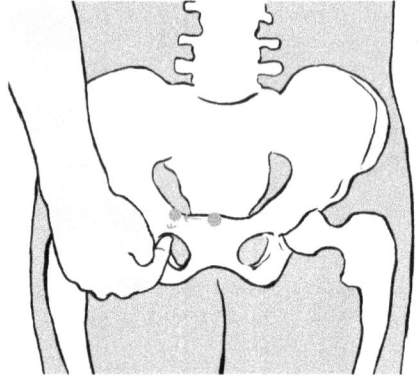

Page 38. Tender Points

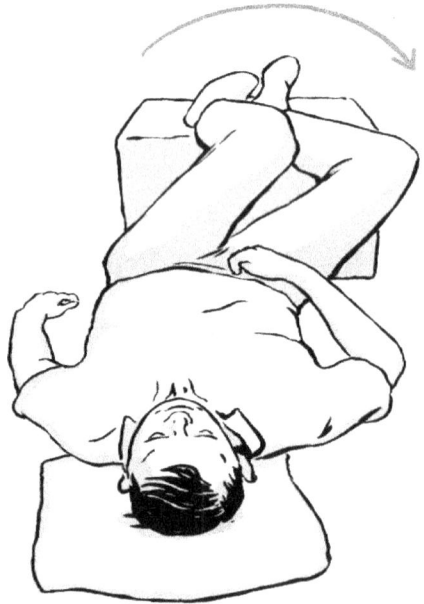

Page 41. Positional Release

Oblique (Lower)

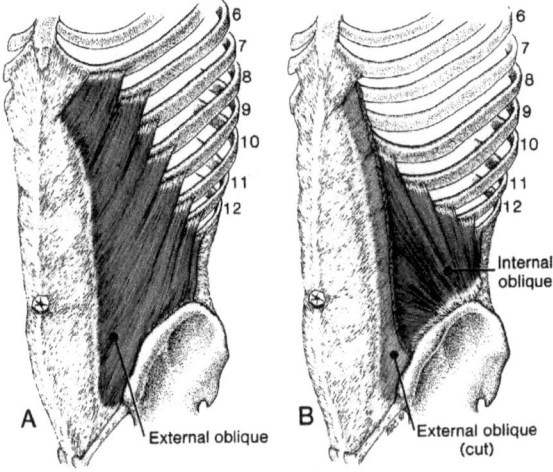

A — External oblique

B — External oblique (cut), Internal oblique

Page 45. Oblique (Lower), L2

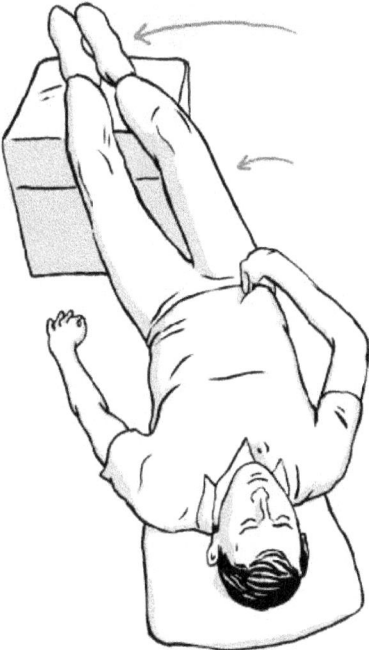

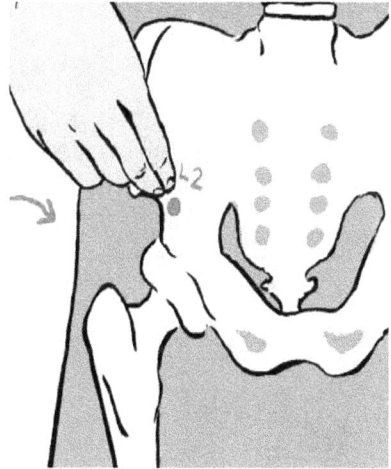

Page 52. Tender Points

Page 55. Positional Release

Iliacus (Lower)

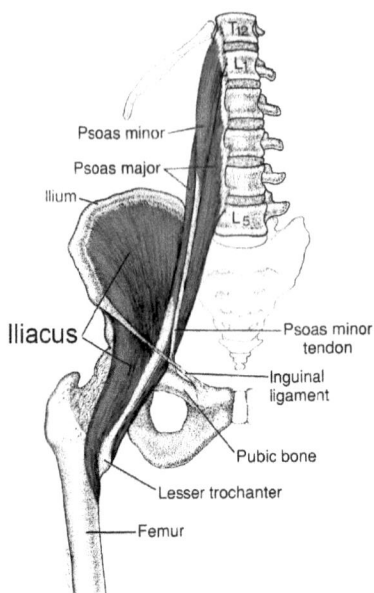

Page 59. Iliacus (Lower), L3, L4

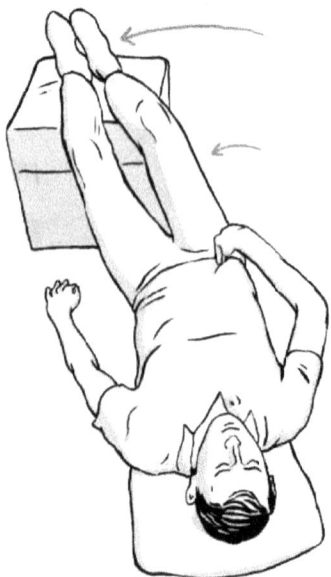

Page 66, 68. Tender Points

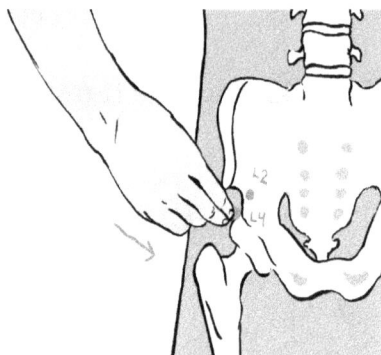

Page 72. Positional Release

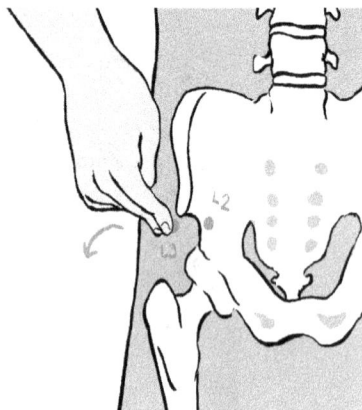

Oblique (Upper)

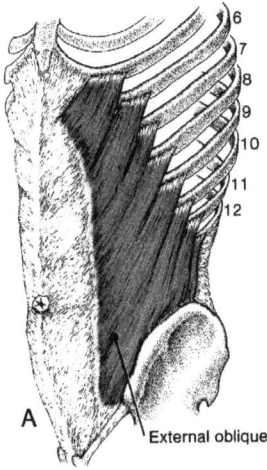

Page 83. Oblique (Upper)

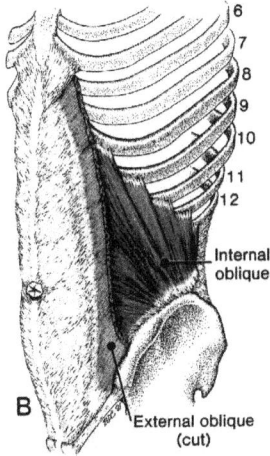

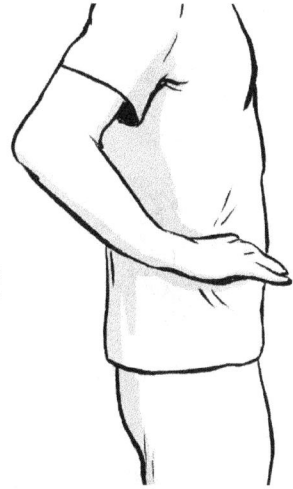

Page 87. Tender Points

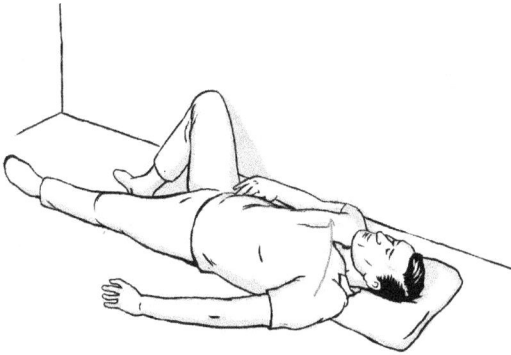

Page 92. Positional Release (Option 1)

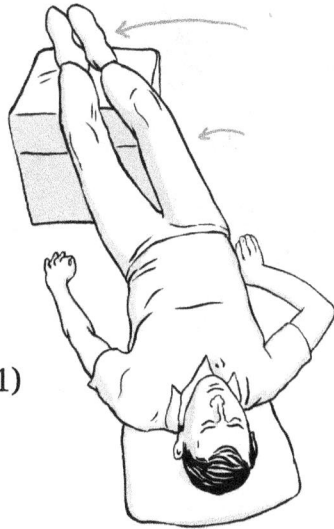

Page 101. Positional Release (Option 2)

Spinal

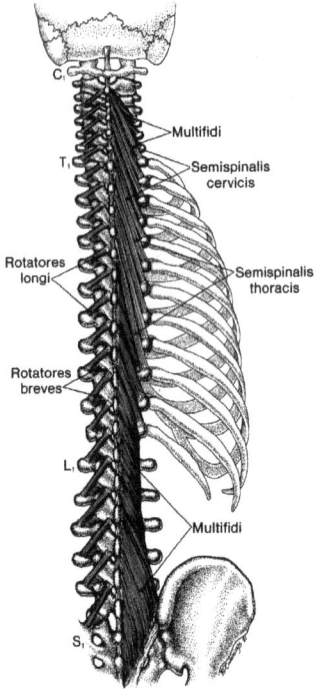

Page 105. Spinal

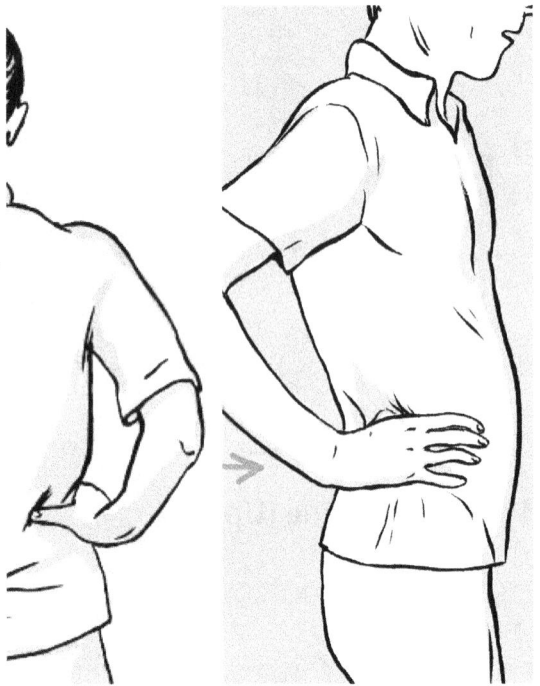

Page 112, 113. Tender Points

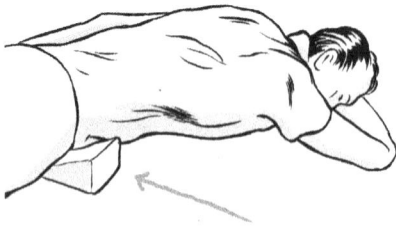

Page 119. Positional Release (Option 1)

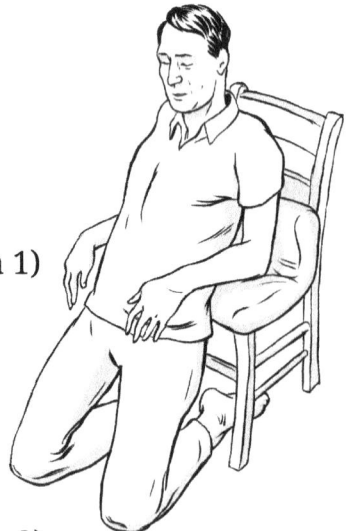

Page 124. Positional Release (Option 2)

Quadratus Lumborum

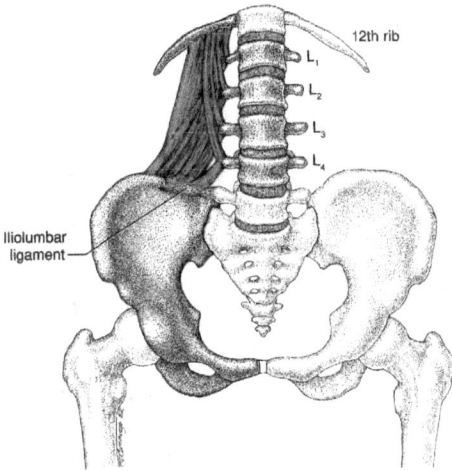

Page 127. Quadratus Lumborum

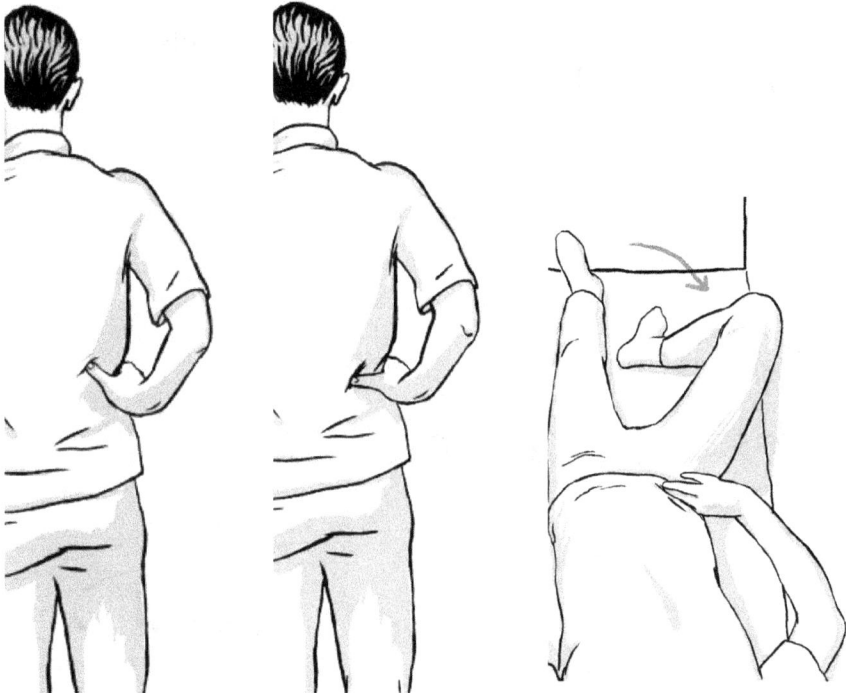

Page 131, 132. Tender Points   Page 135. Positional Release

Piriformis

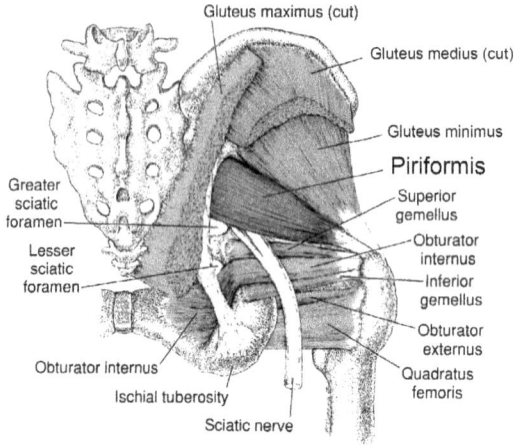

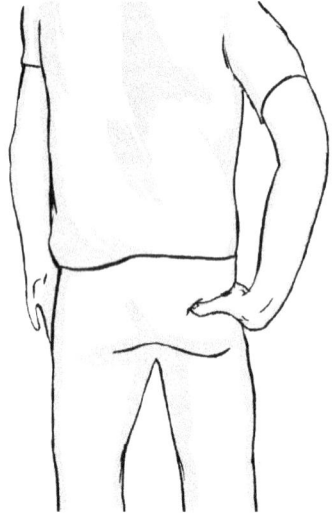

Page 141. Piriformis

Page 145. Tender Points

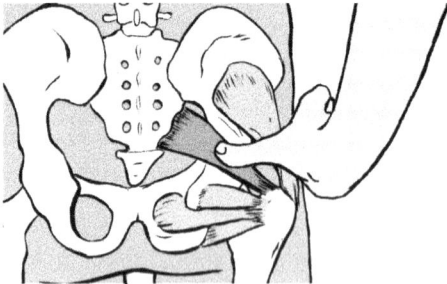

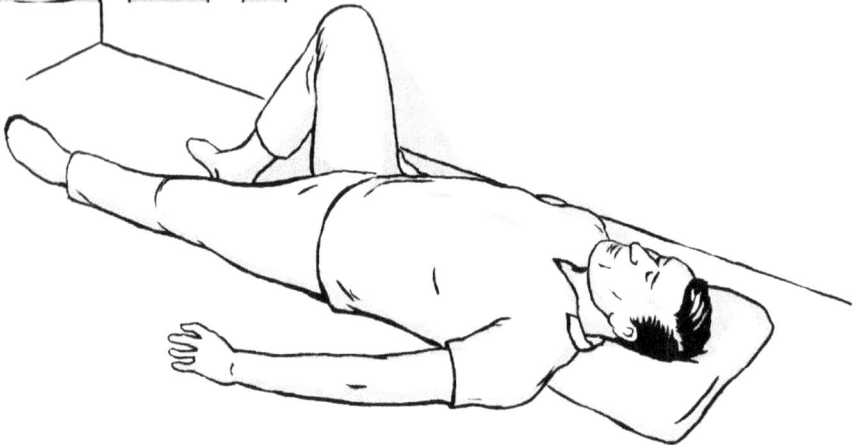

Page 150. Positional Release